Spiritual Assessment in
Healthcare Practice

Other Health and Social Care books from M&K Publishing include:

Nurses and Their Patients:
Informing practice through psychodynamic insights
ISBN: 978-1-905539-31-4 · 2009

Research Issues in Health and Social Care
ISBN: 978-1-905539-20-8 · 2009

Perspectives on Death and Dying
ISBN: 978-1-905539-21-5 · 2009

Identification and Treatment of Alcohol Dependency
ISBN: 978-1-905539-16-1 · 2008

Inter-professional Approaches to Young Fathers
ISBN: 978-1-905539-29-1 · 2008

The Clinician's Guide to Chronic Disease Management
for Long Term Conditions: A cognitive-behavioural approach
ISBN: 978-1-905539-15-4 · 2008

The ECG Workbook
ISBN: 978-1-905539-14-7 · 2008

Routine Blood Results Explained (2nd edition)
ISBN: 978-1-905539-38-3 · 2007

Improving Patient Outcomes
ISBN: 978-1-905539-06-2 · 2007

The Management of COPD in Primary and Secondary Care
ISBN: 978-1-905539-28-4 · 2007

Pre-Teen and Teenage Pregnancy:
A twenty-first century reality
ISBN: 978-1-905539-11-6 · 2007

Issues in Heart Failure Nursing
ISBN: 978-1-905539-00-0 · 2006

Spiritual Assessment in Healthcare Practice

Edited by Wilfred McSherry and Linda Ross

With a foreword by Dr Androulla Johnstone

Spiritual Assessment in Healthcare Practice
Wilfred McSherry and Linda Ross

ISBN: 978-1-905539-27-7

First published 2010

100631858 7

British Library Cataloguing in Publication Data
A catalogue record for this book is available from the British Library

Notice
Clinical practice and medical knowledge constantly evolve. Standard safety precautions must be followed, but, as knowledge is broadened by research, changes in practice, treatment and drug therapy may become necessary or appropriate. Readers must check the most current product information provided by the manufacturer of each drug to be administered and verify the dosages and correct administration, as well as contraindications. It is the responsibility of the practitioner, utilising the experience and knowledge of the patient, to determine dosages and the best treatment for each individual patient. Any brands mentioned in this book are as examples only and are not endorsed by the publisher. Neither the publisher nor the authors assume any liability for any injury and/or damage to persons or property arising from this publication.

To contact M&K Publishing write to:
M&K Update Ltd · The Old Bakery · St. John's Street
Keswick · Cumbria CA12 5AS
Tel: 01768 773030 · Fax: 01768 781099
publishing@mkupdate.co.uk
www.mkupdate.co.uk

Designed and typeset in 11pt Usherwood Book by Mary Blood
Printed in England by Reeds Pinters, Penrith

Contents

Foreword

I was delighted to be asked to provide the foreword for this book. *Spiritual Assessment in Healthcare Practice* provides an arena for both action and debate. It provides a current and in-depth picture of how spirituality is perceived within healthcare provision and offers a vision of how practitioners can work realistically with patients and users of their services.

Over the past 30 years I have observed many fundamental changes in the way that spirituality is integrated into the provision of healthcare. In the late 1970s and early 1980s every hospital had a traditional chaplaincy service and a designated place of worship. The chaplaincy was placed in a senior position within the hospital hierarchy and could be viewed as the vanguard of cultural diversity in healthcare because they were quick to embrace multi-faith worship and spirituality in their services. The notion of a spiritual community was not considered to be out of place within health provision. All kinds of people – patients, staff and carers – observed the human rights of passage – birth, marriage and death – within the boundaries of hospital walls. Spirituality was not something to either dismiss or be 'politically correct' about. However, today, spirituality in healthcare can struggle to find its place in busy provider scenarios where patients are often moved rapidly through the system, living within a society that maintains a growing ambivalence towards matters concerning faith. This book offers the practitioner room to pause for thought and an opportunity to consider new ways of looking at this issue.

When commending this book to readers it is impossible not to consider the media outpourings regarding the current confusion within society when considering spirituality in healthcare. It is not uncommon to read about healthcare professionals who have been criticised for attempting to reach out and provide a spiritual aspect to the care they have provided to patients. The seeming ever-present constraint to provide services that are deemed inoffensive, politically correct, and almost neutral in nature can provide a difficult environment in which to consider spiritual need. The strength of this book is that it presents the conceptual, practical, organisational and ethical challenges that face every healthcare practitioner. The implications of providing spiritual assessment are examined and discussed in a sure-footed manner. The first three chapters provide both a context and a narrative for the reader that affords a unique opportunity for reflection.

It is also impossible to ignore the fact that for the past 30 years 'spirituality' has been a requirement of holistic patient assessment. Yet it is still rare to find documented assessments of spirituality within a patient's record. Most often the section marked 'spirituality' is annotated with a tokenistic demarcation like 'Jewish', 'Catholic' or 'Muslim'. Such labels rarely lead to a more in-depth consideration or plan of care. *Spiritual Assessment in Healthcare Practice* not only presents a clear challenge, but also provides both practical advice and the tools required to equip healthcare practitioners to undertake that challenge. The later chapters in the book examine the numerous practical considerations and set out clear, well-researched and robust strategies for practitioners to apply in their field.

This book sensibly provides a current and in-depth picture of how spirituality is perceived within healthcare provision. It gives the reader an opportunity to examine his or her own notions of spirituality when set within the context of clinical practice. It provides a comprehensive breakdown of what spirituality means within our current society. The final chapter neatly links the concept of spirituality with that of dignity and reflects upon the experience being offered to many patients and users of services today. It also invites us to consider the care that we give in the context of compassion, humanity and sensitivity to the needs of others.

Spiritual Assessment in Healthcare Practice is a satisfying blend of academic research, professional debate and practical assessment strategy. It exhorts the reader to move away from the sidelines and to become involved in the agenda. The default position of 'Do nothing' is successfully challenged and thus opens up new opportunities for practitioners and places the humanity of the patient and service user at the centre of the assessment process.

Dr Androulla Johnstone
CEO of The Health and Social Care Advisory Service (HASCAS)

Contributors

Donia Baldacchino PhD(Hull), MSc(Lond), BSc(Hons), Cert. Ed.(Lond), RGN
Senior Lecturer and Co-ordinator of the MSc Nursing/Midwifery Programme
Institute of Health Care, University of Malta and Visiting Fellow at the University of
Glamorgan, Wales, UK

Donia completed her PhD in 2002 by undertaking a longitudinal study on spiritual coping strategies, anxiety, depression and spiritual well-being of patients with first myocardial infarction. Since then she has published widely on the subject. She is currently coordinating various research studies locally and in collaboration with overseas universities on students' stress and spiritual coping, nursing and caring. She is also exploring stress and spiritual coping in patients with cancer, HIV and AIDS, and institutionalised older persons.

Mark Cobb BSc, MA
Senior Chaplain and Clinical Director
Sheffield Teaching Hospitals NHS Foundation Trust (UK), Sheffield, UK

Mark works in the context of acute healthcare and has specialised in supportive and palliative care. He has a particular interest in the relationship of spirituality to health and well-being which he has explored through practical theology and the sociology of religion. Much of his research activity and teaching is multidisciplinary but he also contributes to developing the practice and profession of healthcare chaplaincy.

Chris Johnson MA (Leeds)
Chaplaincy Manager and Church of England Chaplain
Bradford Teaching Hospitals NHS Trust, Bradford, UK

Chris is currently working on his PhD thesis looking at healthcare staff's understanding and practice of spiritual care assessment of patients in the acute setting. This work involves considering staff's knowledge of spiritual assessment tools within care plans and where necessary developing new tools to assist with these assessments.

Wilfred McSherry PhD, MPhil, BSc(Hons), PGCE(FE), PGCRM, RGN, NT, ILTM
Professor in Dignity of Care for Older People
Staffordshire University and Shrewsbury and Telford Hospital NHS Trust, Stafford and Shrewsbury, UK

Wilf was appointed Professor in Dignity of Care for Older People in August 2008. His interest in the spiritual dimension developed alongside a realisation that this aspect of care was neglected and forgotten by some healthcare professionals. He has published books and articles addressing different aspects of the spiritual dimension. He completed his doctoral studies at Leeds Metropolitan University in May 2005 researching 'The meaning of spirituality and spiritual care: An investigation of healthcare professionals', patients' and public's perceptions'. Prior to being appointed to his current role, Wilf was a senior lecturer in nursing at the University of Hull where he was also instrumental in creating with colleagues the Centre for Spirituality Studies of which he was the director.

Aru Narayanasamy BA, MSc, MPhil, PhD, RN (Adult and Mental Health), FHEA, National Teaching Fellowship
Associate Professor/Theme Leader (Ethnic Diversity and Spirituality)
University of Nottingham, Nottingham, UK

Aru teaches ethnicity, diversity and spiritual health in the School of Nursing, Midwifery and Physiotherapy at the University of Nottingham. He holds the prestigious National Teaching Fellowship awarded by the UK Higher Education Academy for his outstanding work on spirituality and cultural diversity. His pioneering work culminated in teaching innovations such as the ASSET (Actioning Spirituality and Spiritual Care Education and Training) and ACCESS (Transcultural) models.

Christina Puchalski MD FACP OCDS

Board-certified internist and palliative care physician, Founder and Executive Director of the George Washington Institute for Spirituality and Health and Professor of Medicine and Health Sciences at the George Washington University School of Medicine.

Christina is an active clinician, board-certified in Internal Medicine and Palliative Care. In addition to her work on the editorial boards of several palliative care journals, serving as principal or co-principal investigator in numerous research projects, and speaking about spirituality and medicine at national and international conferences, Christina has authored numerous chapters in books as well as writing two books, the first published by Oxford University Press entitled *Time for Listening and Caring: Spirituality and the Care of the Seriously Ill and Dying* with a foreword by His Holiness the Dalai Lama, and the second entitled *Making Healthcare Whole: Integrating Spirituality into Patient Care* published by The Templeton Press, which describes a consensus-derived model and recommendations for interprofessional spiritual care.

Linda Ross BA Nursing (Commendation), RGN, PhD

Senior Lecturer
Department of Care Sciences, Faculty of Health, Sport and Science, University of Glamorgan, Wales, UK

Linda has dedicated most of her career to researching and publishing on spiritual aspects of healthcare. Her PhD thesis on nurses' perceptions of spiritual care was the first study of its kind and size and it is widely quoted. Her post-doctoral work has explored elderly patients' perceptions of their spiritual needs and care and her current work focuses on the spiritual needs and preferences of end-stage heart failure sufferers and their families. She has published widely on spiritual aspects of healthcare including a book entitled *Spiritual Aspects of Nursing* published by Avebury in 1997. She regularly presents her work at conferences and leads workshops for healthcare staff both in the UK and abroad. Educating nurses to provide spiritual care is a further aspect of Linda's teaching, research and writing.

John Swinton PhD, BD, RNMH, RMN
Professor in Practical Theology and Pastoral Care
University of Aberdeen, Aberdeen, Scotland, UK

John is a dual-trained registered nurse who has specialised in psychiatry and learning disabilities. He also worked for a number of years as a community mental health chaplain. His areas of research include the relationship between spirituality and health and the theology and spirituality of disability. In 2004 Professor Swinton founded the Centre for Spirituality, Health and Disability at the University of Aberdeen (http://www.abdn.ac.uk/cshad). He has published widely in the areas of spirituality and health and the theology of disability. His most recent book is *Raging with Compassion: Pastoral Responses to the Problem of Evil* published by Eerdmans in 2007) and he co-authored *Practical Theology and Qualitative Research* by SCM Press in 2006.

Introduction
Linda Ross and Wilfred McSherry

Clearly there has been a groundswell of interest in and recognition of the importance that the spiritual dimension of a person plays in their recovery from illness and in the attainment and maintenance of health, well-being and quality of life.

This has inevitably resulted in healthcare professionals seeking to incorporate spiritual care into their practice. In the past few years, in particular, the authors have become increasingly aware of healthcare professionals (including chaplains, nurses, occupational therapists, physiotherapists, doctors and social workers) asking how they might include the spiritual dimension in their assessment of patients/clients.

The editors are aware that in places the book draws heavily on the nursing literature and practice; however this is not to exclude other disciplines but rather it is a reflection of the pioneering work that has been undertaken by nurses in this area. Increasingly the focus on the spiritual has been taken further, with many other professions developing spiritual assessment and audit tools to assist them in this quest as well as responding to demands for transparency and accountability from management. This has resulted in a mesmerising selection of assessment and audit tools. Some of these are published, while many are not, although they are being used routinely in practice. Informal discussion with some chaplaincy departments reveals that assessment tools, once used, are being replaced by less formal forms of assessment, often using a series of questions as prompts to give patients/clients permission to discuss spiritual matters.

It is against this backdrop that we felt it timely to compile this book on spiritual assessment within healthcare. It is a collection of work that offers insight into this important topic from eminent people in the field. It is not intended to be read from cover to cover, rather it is a resource to be tapped into. Each eminent contributor writes in his or her own unique style and offers insight from their own perspective at this point in time. Some chapters are interactive in their approach while others are more academic. There is also some degree of overlap between the chapters, which enables each chapter to stand alone.

We start, in the first chapter, by asking why spirituality and spiritual care have come to the fore within healthcare in recent years, assuming increasing importance, attention and media interest. But what does the term 'spirituality' actually mean? Rather than attempt to define the concept, as has been done in numerous texts and papers before, the different approaches to spirituality as they apply to the way people live their lives and perceive the world around them are presented in Chapter 2. This sets the scene then for Chapter 3 to consider how, when people face illness, we as healthcare practitioners might recognise signs of spiritual need or distress. Chapters 4 and 5 then focus on how the spiritual dimension might be included within our assessment of the 'whole' person so that the spiritual resources that are part of the patient's everyday life, or perhaps come to the fore for the first time in the face of crisis, are not overlooked in their recovery from and/or adjustment to illness.

Having highlighted that the subject of spirituality has been the focus of considerable research in recent years, the different tools and instruments used to measure spirituality and spiritual well-being (or distress) that contribute to an emerging evidence base for spirituality within healthcare are considered in Chapter 6. Inevitably any attempt to address such a sensitive and deeply personal part of a person's life will attract criticism and debate as highlighted by recent media coverage. Some of the dilemmas faced by healthcare practitioners in attempting to include the spiritual part of the person within a holistic assessment are considered in Chapter 7. Finally, in a health service where the quality of care and treatment features high on the agenda, Chapter 8 focuses on how the quality of spiritual care might be measured.

In the concluding chapter (Chapter 9) we attempt to bring together the main issues raised by all of the contributors and to return to the most important person at the heart of our health service – the patient. We therefore return to the central concern in all of the preceding discussion and debate: how can we as healthcare practitioners best address the spiritual concerns of our patients so that they are assisted to achieve an optimum state of health and well-being? We offer a model for actioning spiritual care and for integrating spiritual assessment within that process. The model is uncannily reminiscent of our early work in this field almost two decades ago, raising questions and challenges for us as to what has actually changed in that time. It remains for us to reflect upon that and we hope that this book offers you, the reader, the opportunity for similar reflection. In that quest we hope you find this contribution useful.

Chapter 1
Why the increasing interest in spirituality within healthcare?

Linda Ross

Introduction

This chapter asks why spiritual care and spiritual assessment have come to the fore within healthcare in recent years. The drivers responsible for the increase in attention given to spiritual matters within healthcare in the UK will be explored by looking at changes in society, as well as healthcare policy and guidelines for professional practice.

Historical perspective

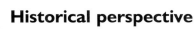

Historical perspective

Most ancient civilisations were aware of the importance of the phenomena, other than those that were directly observable, in influencing illness and disease; religious belief or faith was one such phenomenon. Ancient western philosophers such as Plato recognised the importance of treating people as whole beings – body, mind and spirit:

> *There are physicians for the body and physicians for the soul yet the two are one and indivisible.*
>
> Plato, cited in Grubb, 1977, p. 33

Historically in the West, medical and nursing care were delivered within religious orders where body and soul were regarded as being inseparably linked (e.g. the Knights Hospitallers of St John (Ross, 1997). However, following the 'period of enlightenment' in the eighteenth century, with the escalation in medical research and knowledge, care of the body and soul became separated. Greater emphasis was placed on disease processes and treatments that relied heavily on objective, measurable data and the attention given to the soul declined. Thus the biomedical model emerged with its focus on the physical processes of disease. It failed to acknowledge the important part that other factors, such as the psychological, spiritual, social and individual, have on disease and illness.

Although the medical model is still prevalent in modern day healthcare, the last 50 years have witnessed increasing attempts to return to and re-discover a more holistic approach to care, recognising that the human being is more than a set of physical processes. This holistic approach acknowledges the interplay of the mind, body and spirit where the whole is greater than the sum of the individual parts. One example is the hospice movement. While the word 'hospice' was first coined in the fourth century by Christian orders looking after the varied needs of weary travellers, it was first applied to care of the dying by Madame Jeanne Garnier who founded the Dames de Calaire in Lyon in France in 1842. The name was then used by the Irish Sisters of Charity when they opened Our Lady's Hospice in Dublin in 1879 and by St Joseph's Hospice in London in 1905. Dame Cicely Saunders, who had worked in St Joseph's, went on to found the world-renowned St Christopher's Hospice in 1967, where the focus of care was on mind, body and spirit. This holistic focus is also the sentiment embodied in the Hippocratic Oath which is still sworn by doctors today as a rite of passage in which they promise to practice medicine ethically.

Re-emergence of the spiritual

Re-emergence of the spiritual

Increasingly within our society the metaphysical is being sought after as people yearn for something more to life than the purely physical. Bookshops have ever-growing sections dedicated to spirituality. One high-street store has a section entitled 'Mind, body and spirit' that covers topics such as the occult, mind over matter, crystals and horoscopes. Newspaper and magazine articles regularly focus on the metaphysical, featuring articles on faith healing, the power of the mind over the body, meditation, mystical religions and feng shui, among others. There is also growing recognition of the importance of integrating spiritual principles like mindfulness, connectedness and integrity into the workplace (see http://www.workplacespirituality.org.uk) and within leadership (e.g. Biberman and Tischler, 2008) and education (e.g. Chickering *et al.*, 2006). Social work and social care are acknowledging the increased importance of spirituality within their disciplines too. This is evidenced by the wide array of literature (e.g. Holloway and Moss, 2010), research and other scholarly work that is now taking place (e.g. the International Conference on Spirituality and Social Work, Canada, 2010).

Within the healthcare arena different therapies, such as complementary, music, art, laughter, meditation and relaxation, are gaining more popularity as people recognise the interplay of the mind, body and spirit in their health and well-being. Considerable work is currently being undertaken on spirituality within the mental health sector, such as that by the Royal College of Psychiatrists' Spirituality and Psychiatry Special Interest Group (see http://www.rcpsych.ac.uk/spirit).

Recent media attention has focused on spiritual issues with headlines like 'Nurse sacked for advising patient to go to church' (http://www.nursingtimes.net) and 'A Christian nurse suspended for offering to pray has sparked health care and religion debate' (http://www.nursingtimes.net). The *Nursing Times* reported that the latter story attracted more comments than any other story they had published, indicating that spiritual matters are uppermost in people's minds. Thus, there is more and more recognition within our society in general, and within healthcare in particular, that the metaphysical or spiritual dimension is an important part of life as reflected in policy initiatives, literature, research and other healthcare-related activity, professional legislation and codes of ethics.

Policy initiatives

Global

The recent work of organisations such as the World Health Organization (WHO) emphasises the significance that the spiritual dimension has on health at the world level. Over the years, the WHO has made many statements about the importance of the spiritual part of the person. For example it states:

> Until recently the health professions have largely followed a
> medical model, which seeks to treat patients by focusing on

medicines and surgery, and gives less importance to beliefs and faith. This reductionist or mechanistic view of patients as being only a material body is no longer satisfactory. Patients and physicians have begun to realise the value of elements such as faith, hope and compassion in the healing process. The value of such 'spiritual' elements in health and quality of life has led to research in this field in an attempt to move towards a more holistic view of health that includes a non-material dimension, emphasising seamless connections between mind and body.

NHS Education for Scotland, 2009, p. 7

As far back as 1948 a preamble to the WHO constitution provided this definition:

Health is not just the absence of disease. It is a state of physical, psychological, social and spiritual well-being.

NHS Education for Scotland, 2009, p. 6

More recently the WHO has included spirituality within health impact assessment. Thirty-two questions relating to people's spiritual, religious or personal beliefs and how these impact on their quality of life (QOL) are included in the WHO QOL Spirituality, Religiousness and Personal Beliefs (SRPB) Field-Test Instrument (World Health Organization, 2002). Spirituality also features in the WHO work on palliative care, ageing and disaster relief (http://www.who.int/en). Whether this work results in alteration of the WHO definition of health to include the spiritual, as was suggested in 1948, remains to be seen.

European

At a European level, the Human Rights Act 2000 requires governments to adequately provide for the spiritual and religious needs of their citizens while they are in receipt of healthcare. This requirement has filtered through to the British National Health Service (NHS), where NHS Trusts must provide appropriate world faith representatives and make provision for all faith communities to be able to worship.

National

The Department of Health (DH) is committed, through the NHS Plan (Department of Health, 2000a), to providing services 'around the needs and preferences of individual patients, their families and their carers' irrespective of their 'age, gender, ethnicity, religion, disability or sexuality' (NHS, 2009).

This principle is reflected in *Your Guide to the NHS* thus:

NHS staff will respect your privacy and dignity. They will be sensitive to, and respect your religious, spiritual and cultural needs at all times.

It is also seen in the publication of *The NHS Constitution* (Department of Health, 2009a) where compassionate care is also highlighted. The most recent document *Religion or Belief. A Practical Guide for the NHS* (Department of Health, 2009b) was published to give practical guidance to NHS organisations to meet their responsibilities relating to religion or belief (Department of Health, 2009b).

In addition to these general documents produced by the Department of Health, further guidance is provided for specific groups. For instance, the National Institute for Health and Clinical Excellence's (NICE) guidance entitled *Supportive and Palliative Care for Adults with Cancer* (National Institute for Health and Clinical Excellence, 2004), the Marie Curie's *Spiritual and Religious Care Competencies for Specialist Palliative Care* (Marie Curie Cancer Care, 2003) and the National Service Frameworks (provide national standards for respecting people's privacy, dignity, religious and spiritual beliefs) relate specifically to coronary heart disease, care of the older person, and mental health (Department of Health, 1999, 2000b, 2001b). Further, the concept of dignity is increasingly gaining attention as evidenced by recent government guidance (Social Care Institute for Excellence, 2006) and the Royal College of Nursing's 'Dignity – at the heart of everything we do' campaign (Royal College of Nursing, 2008).

The value that our NHS places on spiritual care is further reflected in its employment of hospital chaplains who are paid to minister to the religious and non-religious spiritual needs of patients and staff. The provision of spiritual and religious care has been a part of the NHS since its inception in 1948. Guidance for the provision of chaplaincy and spiritual care services has responded to changes in the needs of society over time. The most recent guidance (Department of Health, 2003) seeks to enable chaplaincy and spiritual care services to meet the needs of today's increasingly multicultural and spiritually diverse society. It replaces previous guidance by the NHS Executive (1995), the National Association of Health Authorities and Trusts (1996) and responds to the Human Rights Act 2000 requirements as outlined above.

In Scotland, all fourteen NHS Boards have developed their own spiritual care policies, and all Trusts have action plans in place to meet policy objectives. The most recent spiritual care revised guidance requires Chief Executives to appoint senior lead managers for spiritual care, to update existing policy and ensure adequate resourcing for the provision of a twenty-four hour spiritual care/chaplaincy service (Scottish Government, 2009). Considerable education opportunities also exist for staff (NHS Education for Scotland, 2009).

Healthcare literature, research and other related activity

Healthcare literature

Within the general body of healthcare literature there has been a rapid increase in recent years in the number of articles referring to the spiritual dimension of care. These articles have raised awareness of and initiated debate on the spiritual dimension within healthcare from the disciplines of medicine, nursing and the professions allied to medicine (PAMS) including chaplaincy. For example a recent literature search conducted by the author for the search terms '(spiritual or spiritual care) and nursing' identified 1420 sources in the form of theses, books, chapters in books, letters, editorials, videos, conference abstracts and journal articles.

Focusing specifically on the research, there is a growing body of scientific literature that supports the assertion that the spiritual dimension has significant mental and physical health effects (e.g. Hollywell and Walker, 2008; Koenig *et al.*, 2001; Mental Health Foundation, 2006; Walsh *et al.*, 2002). A systematic review is currently underway for the Cochrane Collaboration examining spiritual and religious interventions for adults in the terminal phase of disease (Candy *et al.*, 2009).

There is also more research on spiritual care within nursing. When this author undertook a literature search during the late 1980s and early 1990s, no UK nursing research studies had been published on spirituality, and only two unpublished small-scale studies were identified (Chomicz, 1984; Simsen, 1988). Most of the North American research was also unpublished (Chance, 1967;

Hitchens, 1988; Kealey, 1974; Kramer, 1957; Lewis, 1957; Piles, 1986). Only one full, published paper was identified (Highfield and Cason, 1983), because most were in a summarised form. When this review was repeated in 2006, 47 original nursing research papers were identified (Ross, 2006) from the UK, the USA, Japan, Australia and across Europe and Scandinavia. This contribution does not include the work being undertaken currently by nurses and other healthcare professionals for higher degrees or the numerous undergraduates conducting literature reviews or small-scale research studies on the subject as part of their degrees.

It is encouraging that many disciplines involved in caring for patients or clients in the NHS, both in practice and in academia, are coming together to share experiences and insights and to be involved in debate on the topic of spiritual care. This is evidenced by the number of study days being held (e.g. Motol Hospital, Prague, 20–23 May 2007; Craiova, Romania, 7–8 October 2005), as well as national conferences e.g. Challenges of Spiritual Care: Theory and Practice, Palliative Care Research Society Conference, London, January 2007; *Nursing Standard*'s Spirit of Nursing Conference, London, April 2009 and international conferences (International Conference on Spirituality and Social Work, Canada, June 2010; Spirituality in a Changing World, Windsor, May 2010); research groups (e.g. European Network of Research on Religion, Spirituality and Health); centres for spirituality (e.g. Universities of Aberdeen, Hull, Staffordshire); and moves toward collaborative working e.g. collaborative research bids, establishment of the British Association for the Study of Spirituality (BASS) which seeks to foster 'further study of spirituality in its practice and theoretical aspects' as well as to 'strengthen teaching and learning of spirituality as an academic and professional discipline' http://www.basspirituality.org.uk).

Professional legislation and codes of ethics

Professional legislation

The spiritual principles of social justice, human dignity and worth are at the heart of codes of ethics – either implicitly or explicitly – of most disciplines in healthcare (e.g. social work, physiotherapy, occupational therapy, medicine). However, within nursing this is taken a step further in that it is explicitly stated that nurses are expected to be involved in the delivery of spiritual care. Florence Nightingale, one of the earliest pioneers of nursing, considered 'the sick body ... is something more than a reservoir for storing medicines' (Kramer, 1957, p. 36). One of the early models of nursing developed by Henderson considered it the duty of the nurse to assist the patient to 'worship according to his faith' (p. 13) and 'practice his religion or conform to his concept of right and wrong' (Henderson, 1977, p. 19). Spirituality is at the heart of other nursing models and theories and is discussed more fully elsewhere (Ross, 1997; McSherry, 2006).

Spiritual care is also central to nursing codes of ethics, both internationally and within the UK. The International Council of Nurses *Code of Ethics for Nurses* states:

> *In providing care, the nurse promotes an environment in which the human rights, values, customs and spiritual beliefs of the individual, family and community are respected.*
>
> International Council of Nurses, 2006, p. 2

In the UK, the NMC Code of Professional Conduct states that:

> *You must treat people as individuals and respect their dignity.*
>
> Nursing and Midwifery Council, 2008, p. 2

The NMC further expects that nurses on qualifying are able to:

> *Undertake and document a comprehensive, systematic and accurate nursing assessment of the physical, psychological, social and spiritual needs of patients, clients and communities.*
>
> Nursing and Midwifery Council, 2004, p. 5

The more recent Essential Skills Clusters for pre-registration nursing programmes identifies 'skills that are essential' to be 'a proficient nurse' (Nursing and Midwifery Council, 2007). Included under the 'Care, compassion and communication' cluster is the expectation that the nurse, at the point of registration, will demonstrate sensitivity and cultural competence, and will make 'a holistic and systematic assessment of ... cultural and spiritual needs' and 'develop a comprehensive plan of nursing care, (Nursing and Midwifery Council, 2007, p. 9).

There is a similar expectation of the Quality Assurance Agency for Higher Education (Quality Assurance Agency, 2001, pp. 10, 12) which expects nurses to be educated to:

- *undertake a comprehensive systematic assessment using the tools/frameworks appropriate to the patient/client taking into account relevant … spiritual needs*
- *plan care delivery to meet identified needs*
- *demonstrate an understanding of issues related to spirituality.*

Respect for the religious and spiritual beliefs of patients/clients is also central to codes of ethics in other countries like the Netherlands, Norway and Malta. The extent to which nurses are taught about spiritual care is, however, variable and it is often dependent upon the interest or expertise of the lecturers within the various university departments. This means that some nurses receive teaching on spiritual care during their basic preparation, but others do not. For those who have received input, the content, amount and delivery will vary. Yet despite these inconsistencies, there is evidence that the teaching of spiritual care is gaining more attention. Increasing numbers of articles are now appearing that describe the teaching that is taking place in different university departments, debating the many issues involved and dilemmas raised and highlighting the need for the development of competencies for spiritual care (Baldacchino, 2006; van Leeuwen and Cusveller, 2004; van Leeuwen *et al.*, 2009). In addition, medical students in some universities in the UK and the USA are now receiving education on spirituality and there are moves to repeat and expand this input within other countries, for example through the work of partnerships in international medical education.

Conclusion

This short chapter attempts to offer some explanation for the increase in the interest in spirituality within healthcare in recent years. One of the main drivers is undoubtedly the influence of healthcare policy, not just nationally, but internationally. This combined with professional legislation and other related activity within the healthcare arena, as well as an increasing awareness of the metaphysical within society at large, has resulted in spiritual care securing a central place within healthcare provision.

References

Baldacchino, D, (2006). 'Nursing competencies for spiritual care'. *Journal of Clinical Nursing,* 15, 885–96.

Biberman, J. and Tischler, L. (2008). *Spirituality in Business. Theory, Practices and Future Directions*. Basingstoke: Palgrave Macmillan.

Candy, B., Jones, L., Speck, P., Tookman, A. and King, M. (2009). *Spiritual and religious interventions for adults in terminal phase of disease (protocol)*. Cochrane Collaboration. London: John Wiley.

Chance, J.P.L. (1967). *Nurses' responses to patients' spiritual needs*. Master's thesis. California: Loma Linda University.

Chickering, A., Dalton, C. and Stamm, L. (2006). *Encouraging Authenticity and Spirituality in Higher Education*. San Francisco: Jossey-Bass.

Chomicz, L. (1984). *What are patients' spiritual needs?* BSc dissertation. London: City University.

Department of Health (1999). *National Service Framework for Mental Health: Modern Standards and Service Models*. London: The Stationery Office.

Department of Health (2000a). *A Plan for Investment, a Plan for Reform*. London: Department of Health.

Department of Health (2000b). *Coronary Heart Disease: National Service Framework for Coronary Heart Disease – Modern Standards and Service Models*. London: The Stationery Office.

Department of Health (2001a). *Your Guide to the NHS*. London: The Stationery Office.

Department of Health (2001b). *National Service Framework for Older People*. London: The Stationery Office.

Department of Health (2003). *NHS Chaplaincy. Meeting the Religious and Spiritual Needs of Patients and Staff*. London: The Stationery Office.

Department of Health (2009a). *The NHS Constitution*. London: The Stationery Office.

Department of Health (2009b). *Religion or Belief. A Practical Guide for the NHS*. London: The Stationery Office.

Grubb, G. (1977). 'The pastor's role in visiting the sick'. *Nursing Mirror*, 144, 33.

Henderson, V. (1977). *Basic Principles of Nursing Care*. Geneva: ICN.

Highfield, M. and Cason, C. (1983). Spiritual needs of patients: Are they recognised? *Cancer Nursing*, 6, 187–92.

Hitchens, E.W. (1988). *Stages of faith and values development and their implications for dealing with spiritual care in the student nurse–patient relationship*. EEd thesis. Seattle: University of Seattle.

Holloway, M. and Moss, B. (2010). *Spirituality and Social Work*. Basingstoke, Palgrave Macmillan.

Hollywell, C. and Walker, J. (2008). 'Private prayer as suitable intervention for hospitalised patients: A critical review of the literature'. *Journal of Clinical Nursing*, 18, 637–51.

International Council of Nurses (2006). *The ICN Code of Ethics for Nurses*. ICN, Geneva.

Kealey, C. (1974). *The patient's perspective on spiritual needs*. Master's thesis. Columbia, University of Missouri.

Koenig, H.G., McCullough, M.E. and Larson, D.B. (2001). *Handbook of Religion and Health*. Oxford and New York: Oxford University Press.

Kramer, P. (1957). *A survey to determine the attitudes and knowledge of a selected group of professional nurses concerning spiritual care of the patient*. Master's thesis. Oregon: University of Oregon.

Lewis, J.E. (1957). *A resource unit on spiritual aspects of nursing for the basic nursing curriculum of a selected school of nursing*. Master's thesis. Seattle: University of Washington.

Marie Curie Cancer Care (2003). *Spiritual and Religious Care Competencies for Specialist Palliative Care*. London: Marie Curie.

McSherry, W. (2006). *Making Sense of Spirituality in Nursing and Health Care Practice*, 2nd edn. London: Jessica Kingsley Publishers.

Mental Health Foundation (2006). *The Impact of Spirituality on Mental Health. A Review of the Literature*. London: Mental Health Foundation.

National Association of Health Authorities and Trusts (1996). *Spiritual Care in the NHS*. Birmingham: NAHAT.

National Institute for Health and Clinical Excellence (2004). *Improving Supportive and Palliative Care for Adults with Cancer*. London: NICE.

NHS (2009). *NHS Core Principles*. Available at: http://www.nhs.uk/NHSEngland/aboutnhs/Pages/NHSCorePrinciples.aspx (last accessed April 2010).

NHS Education for Scotland (2009). *Spiritual Care Matters. An Introductory Resource for all NHS Scotland Staff*. Edinburgh: NES.

NHS Executive (1995). *Framework for Spiritual, Faith and Related Pastoral Care*. Leeds: The Institute of Nursing.

Nursing and Midwifery Council (2004). *Standards of Proficiency for Pre-Registration Nursing Education*. London: NMC.

Nursing and Midwifery Council (2007). *Essential skills clusters (ESCs) for pre-registration nursing programmes. NMC Circular 07/2007*. London: NMC.

Nursing and Midwifery Council (2008). *The Code*. London: NMC.

Piles, C.L. (1986). *Spiritual care: Role of nursing education and practice. A needs survey for curriculum development*. PhD thesis. Saint Louis, MI: University of Saint Louis.

Quality Assurance Agency for Higher Education (2001). *Benchmark Statement: Healthcare Programmes*. Gloucester: QAAHE.

Roper, N., Logan, W. and Tierney, A. (1990) *The Elements of Nursing: A Model for Nursing Based on a Model of Living*, 3rd edn. Churchill Livingstone, Edinburgh.

Ross, L.A. (1997). *Nurses' Perceptions of Spiritual Care*. Aldershot: Avebury.

Ross, L.A. (2006). 'Spiritual care in nursing: An overview of the research to date'. *Journal of Clinical Nursing*, 15(7), 852–62.

Royal College of Nursing (2008). 'RCN launches major campaign on dignity'. *RCN Bulletin*, **204**, 1.

Scottish Executive Health Department (2002). *Guidelines on Chaplaincy and Spiritual Care in the NHS in Scotland*. Available at: http://www.spiritualcare.org.uk/hdl-2002–76.htm.

Scottish Government (2009). *Spiritual Care and Chaplaincy*. Edinburgh: The Stationery Office.

Simsen, B. (1988). 'Nursing the spirit'. *Nursing Times*, **84**(37), 31–33.

Social Care Institute for Excellence (2006). *Adults' Services Practice Guide. Dignity in Care*. London: SCIE.

Van Leeuwen, R. and Cusveller, B. (2004). Nursing competencies for spiritual care. *Journal of Advanced Nursing*, **48**(3), 234–46.

Van Leeuwen, R, Tiesinga, L.J., Middel, B., Post, D. and Jochemsen, H. (2009). 'The validity and reliability of an instrument to assess nursing competencies in spiritual care'. *Journal of Clinical Nursing*, **18**(20), 1–13.

Walsh, K., King, M., Jones, L., Tookman, A. and Blizard, R. (2002). 'Do spiritual beliefs affect outcome of bereavement: A prospective, cohort study'. *British Medical Journal*, **324**, 1551.

World Health Organization (2002). *WHO-QOL SRPB Field-Test Instrument*. Geneva: WHO. Available at: http:/www.who.int/en (last accessed April 2010).

Chapter 2
The meanings of spirituality: a multi-perspective approach to 'the spiritual'
John Swinton

Introduction

There can be little doubt that spirituality is, to a greater or lesser degree, on the agenda of many of the healthcare professions (Ai, 2001; Chatters, 2000; Cobb and Robshaw, 1998; Dawson, 1997; Kirsh, 1996; Koenig, 1998; Powell, 2003; Reynolds, 2000). At one time it could have been argued that spirituality was the 'forgotten' dimension of healthcare (Swinton, 2001), but the recent plethora of writing and research on spirituality and its relationship with health indicates that the memory of the health and social care professions has well and truly been recovered! That is not to say that everyone is remembering it in the same way, of course. The rich diversity of definitions and understandings of spirituality is indicative of a concept that is either extremely important – or so vague as to be unusable.

I was asked to write a chapter outlining what spirituality is. However, I confess that the more I reflect on the issue of spirituality, the less convinced I am that asking the apparently simple question – what is spirituality? – is necessarily the best way to frame the issue. The area of human experience that the term 'spirituality' has come to represent is far too complicated and important to be captured within any single definition or trite answer. In this chapter I will present a multi-perspective approach to spirituality (exploring spirituality from a variety of perspectives) that recognises the diversity of definitions present within the literature and seeks to offer ways in which we might work effectively within the realm of the spiritual, even in the midst of its plurality.

Approaching spirituality

Approaching spirituality

In setting the context for the models of spiritual assessment described in this book, it will be helpful to lay out a number of approaches to spirituality that might enable practitioners to begin to recognise, assess and work with the area of human experience that is represented by the term 'spirituality'. In the following discussion, I will outline a variety of approaches to spirituality that emerge from reflection on the literature. I use the term 'approach' in a quite particular way. To *approach* something is to move towards it, to draw near to it from a particular angle. You do not grasp a thing in all of its fullness as you approach it. Rather you move closer to it, and as you move closer to it so its shape and form become clearer. However, the knowledge gained from any single approach is determined by the *angle* of approach; the particular angle you approach any entity from is important insofar as it will allow you to see some things, and will preclude you from seeing other things. That being so, the approaches to spirituality outlined below should not be read as discrete and separate entities that have any absolute definitive claim on what spirituality is. Rather they should be viewed as different *approaches* to spirituality – different lenses through which we can gaze upon the phenomenon of spirituality. Each approach overlaps and interacts with the others in interesting and important ways. It is as we learn to understand and appreciate the different approaches that the meaning of spirituality can begin to emerge in any given set of circumstances. The three approaches outlined here are:

- *a generic approach*
- *a biological approach*
- *an approach from religion*.

There may well be other approaches, but these three will hopefully be appropriate as a theoretical foundation for the reflections presented here. By briefly outlining these approaches I hope to lay a conceptual framework which will help to provide a context for the various methods of spiritual assessment that are laid out in this book. I would emphasise that these approaches should not be seen as necessarily separate from one another. In practice they constantly cross and flow together with the rhythm of people's experiences and the changing perceptions of and perspectives on spirituality that emerge within the lived experience of ill people and those who seek to offer care and support.

A generic approach

A generic approach

The generic approach to spirituality seems to be the one most prevalent within the British nursing literature and within legislative definitions of what spirituality is. For something to be considered 'generic' it needs to be applicable to an entire class or group of people. Therefore, for spirituality to be 'generic' it needs to be something that is applicable to all people in all cultures and at all times. Generic spirituality is a form of spirituality that is stripped of any specific tradition – religious or otherwise; it is assumed to be a human universal. Its definition may be fluid, but however it is defined, it is assumed to exist as a human reality that can be formally identified and assessed as a significant dimension of human experience which includes, but is not defined by, religion. A generic approach assumes that spiritual care is for people of 'all faiths and none'.

The advantage of this approach is that carers' attention is drawn to important aspects of the person that might not otherwise be on the caring agenda. In assuming that the person is in essence spiritual, irrespective of their involvement or otherwise in formal religion, issues of meaning, purpose, value, hope and love are brought to the fore. In this way the phenomenology of illness (that is, the meanings that people ascribe to their illness experiences that might be quite different from the medical meanings of their illness) is given priority, thus leading to genuinely person-centred care that respects medicine but is not dictated to by its explanatory frameworks. As such, a generic approach to spirituality has the potential to improve both the standard and the meaningfulness of our caring practices.

Limitations of a purely generic approach

However, the generic approach is not without its difficulties. First, this model does not actually describe what spirituality is. In defining spirituality in such terms as the human search for meaning, hope, love, transcendence, purpose, value connected-ness, and sometimes God, people are describing *spiritual well-being*, meaning the effects of a person's spirituality rather than what *spirituality* – understood as an identifiable, discrete entity – might actually be. The question of what spirituality *does* seems quite clear: it facilitates the attainment of peace, meaning, hope, and so forth. The question of what spirituality *is* remains a mystery. When we try to capture that mystery in language such as 'a connection with the universe', 'the essential life force', or 'that which relates us to all that is around', we find ourselves using language that is very difficult to make sense of in a clinical context. So we try to translate that language into human experiences, which are much more obvious in terms of what we might do with them when we encounter them in our day-to-day duties.

In some ways, while understandable, this tendency to translate the intangible into the tangible is rather an odd and strangely contradictory approach. Many of those who adopt this approach push towards a position which they claim stands against reductionistic materialism. Yet, in the attempt to name and assess spirituality they end up focusing on its *effects*. In other words, they end up turning that which is assumed to be immaterial and transcendent into something that is material and immanent and which, if not directly observable, can at least be made recognis-able in linguistic and experiential terms (i.e. experienced via the material body). So in a strangely materialistic way, those holding this position translate spirituality into the various experiences and embodiments that are in fact the consequence of the outworking of the spirit, rather than ontological, that is, a description of what spirituality actually *is* rather than what it *does*. In translating the experiences that it is argued form a person's spirituality into experiential and material terms, therefore, these theorists end up becoming materialists and empiricists!

Perhaps most importantly, the aspects identified as being definitive of spirituality are not recognised as central to the spiritual-ity of many people, particularly those religions for whom such things as the search for meaning, purpose or transcendence are not central to the way in which they perceive spirituality, such as in Islam and Theravada Buddhism. This means that in the quest for inclusiveness and spiritual correctness (Swinton and Mowat, 2006) there is a danger that one ends up engaging in a rather odd mode of spiritual colonialism that masquerades as spiritual universalism: 'all people have a spirituality and this is what it is!'. It has been noted that when you break down many of the definitions people offer for generic spirituality, they end up looking more like a secularised version of Christianity (Markham, 1998) carried out within an existentialist framework that bears a remarkable resemblance to Victor Frankl's logotherapy, that is, the underlying assumption that the search for meaning is a primary human goal (Frankl, 1997).

I would, however, want to stress that none of this needs to be perceived as a reason for rejecting the generic model of spirituality. Drawing attention to the fact that many people when they encounter illness will begin to ask the big questions in life – Who am I? Where do I come from? Where am I going to? Why? – can only be a useful sensitisation to dimensions of human experience which can easily be lost in an overly materialistic approach to healthcare that separates the physical from the experiential. Again, positively, the recognition that we may well be talking about noticing, measuring and assessing areas of human experience that we have chosen to define as 'spiritual well-being' rather than a thing called 'spirituality', might actually be a way of avoiding or moving beyond the continuing and entrenched discussion about what spirituality actually is or is not – a conversation that is linguistically and philosophically interesting (Paley, 2008) but in the end makes little difference to the lives of the patients we seek to offer effective care to.

The issues raised above simply mean that we need to recognise that the idea of generic spirituality is more complicated than we might at first assume and often does not do what we might think or hope it might do. Problems arise when we uncritically assume that this is the *only* way to understand spirituality.

An approach from biology

A second approach, and one which is often tied in with the generic approach, is the biological approach to spirituality. Put simply, the biological approach proposes that spirituality is present in all human beings for biological and evolutionary purposes; human beings are hard-wired for religious and spiritual experience (Hay, 2006a,b; Newberg *et al.*, 2001). In other words, there is a specific area of the brain that is designed to receive religious and spiritual experiences, in the same way that there are areas of the brain designed to receive sound, vision and so forth. An interesting exemplar of this approach is David Hay's work on what he describes as 'the biology of God' (Hay, 2006a,b). Hay is a zoologist who bases his work on the thinking of the biologist Alasdair Hardy. In his Gifford Lectures, which he presented at the University of Aberdeen (Hardy, 1965), Hardy put forward the thesis that religious experience was present in all human beings for evolutionary purposes. Over many years Hay has developed Hardy's work and has put forward some convincing evidence for there being a biological basis for spiritual experience. In his book *The Spirituality of the Child* (Hay, 2006a,b), Hay proposes that children are naturally spiritual; that they have an inherent sense of awe, wonder and acceptance of things beyond their understanding. This inherent awareness he describes as *relational consciousness*. Relational consciousness is a form of consciousness characterised by the fact that it is always relational: self–other people, self–environment, self–God. Hay argues that this is what makes spirituality possible and in a certain sense 'is' spirituality. Phenomenologically it is experienced as the shortening of the psychological distance between self and the rest of reality; a dissolving of the boundaries, that at the limit becomes the loss of distinction between self and some other, similar to the experience of the mystic. From Hay's perspective this is the source of the experiential basis of religion, seen as a social construction in response to experience.

However, while spirituality is relational and inherent within the experiences of children, when they enter the educational system they become *de-spiritualised*. They are taught to think logically and rationally and to downgrade or even exclude the pre-school spiritual experiences that were so formative of their early years. Hay identifies this spiritual repression with certain forms of frustration and aggression encountered by children in their teens. If we accept Hay's hypotheses, then three important things emerge. First, in opposition to Freudian ideas about the social construction of religion (see the section below on Freud's theory of religion and projection) it is actually *secularisation* that is socially constructed, in opposition to the *natural* human experience of spirituality. Second, if this mode of thinking is correct, then it is not only overtly religious patients that will be experiencing spirituality and spiritual issues, *but* all of the patients whom carers encounter; this gives some added empirical weight to the generic approach. Third, if there is a biological or evolutionary basis for spirituality and spiritual experience, it becomes easier to understand why there might be a connection between spirituality, religion and health. We will explore this connection in more detail below.

This approach is helpful in that, as per the generic approach, it indicates that there is a commonality of certain human needs, which it is important for carers to recognise and to be prepared to work with. In drawing attention to the inherent relationality of human beings, the biological approach offers a perspective about living well that moves us away from individualism and towards community and relationship. This can only be a useful corrective to approaches to care that fragment people and assume them to be individuals without any need for community. Human beings are persons-in-relation (Macmurray, 1961) and this relational dynamic becomes even sharper in times of ill-health when all of us begin to realise that we are in fact dependent rather than individual creatures.

However, locating spirituality within a particular biological structure or structures raises problems. First by stating that spirituality is biological the idea of spirituality is easily reduced to a matter of neurological function alone. There is no need for the transcendent to be real; it simply needs to be perceived as real in order to bring about certain benefits for evolutionary gain. Thus the idea of God or spiritual experience is reduced to a series of synapses within the biology of the brain. Secondly and more importantly, if spirituality has a biological basis, then what happens when that biology is damaged or destroyed through the rigours of ageing, disability or illness? Does the person then become de-spiritualised? Bearing in mind that many definitions of spirituality specifically equate spirituality with the essence of what it means to be human, this approach could be very bad news for people with dementia or brain damage for example. On its own, this approach to spirituality leaves some of our most vulnerable patients even more vulnerable.

On the positive side, this model does give us some insights into the naturalness of human relationality, an aspect of spiritual well-being that tends to unify the various definitions of spirituality within the literature. It also reinforces the important point that certain experiences that we relate to the domain of the spiritual are present in all people. Indeed by reminding us that spirituality at heart has to do with relationships and that caring for relationships is not a secondary task but is fundamentally important to the tasks of caring, the biological approach helps us to overcome the Westernised and colonialist tendencies of the generic approach highlighted previously.

It may well be that spiritual experience has biological correlates, but on its own this approach is inadequate. It requires aspects of the generic approach in order that the specific experiences that it claims make up spirituality are not bound simply by the state of a person's neurology. The generic approach leaves open the possibility that spirituality can be experienced in and through others, including transcendent Others, rather than being bound to any particular aspect of the individual. As such, the two approaches have the potential to be complementary if explored critically and carefully.

Of course, in fairness to David Hay, he would argue that his approach is not reductionist at all. Indeed he would argue that to suggest it was reductionist was to misunderstand the process of evolution. One develops an eye because there is something to see; an ear because there is something to hear; and a spiritual receptor because there is something to receive. That being so, the biological model – at least in some of its manifestations – still leaves open the possibility of the reality of God. Those with a specific interest in religious spirituality may be wary of a biological approach but they needn't necessarily discard it.

An approach from religion

An approach from religion

The approach from religion takes different forms. For ease of analysis we will split it into three basic categories: religion and the transcendent, religion as projection, and religion as behaviour.

Religion and the transcendent

The transcendent approach to religion and religious spirituality begins with the assumption that there is something beyond the self that is the source or the focus of a person's spiritual experiences and spiritual well-being: God or 'transcendence'. This of course is the traditional understanding of spirituality that has underpinned nursing historically (Barnum, 1996). Within this approach carers draw on specific religious traditions and practices to bring about healing and relief (Shelly, Allen and Miller, 1999).

The term 'religion' refers to a formal system of beliefs, which usually centre on some conception of God and express the views of a particular religious group or community. The word 'religion' originates semantically from the Latin word *religio*, a word that 'implies that "foundation wall" to which one is "bound" for one's survival, the basis of one's being' (Sims, 1994, p. 444) More specifically it 'signifies a bond between humanity and some greater-than-human power' (Larson *et al.*, 1997, p. 15). A person's religion, at least in its purest form, is something that is foundational to the way in which they experience themselves and make sense of the world they inhabit. Religion asks deep questions about the nature of human beings, their identity and place within the world, the purpose and meaning of human life, and the destiny of humankind. Organised religions are rooted within a particular tradition or traditions, which engender their own narratives, symbols and doctrines that are used by adherents to interpret and explain their experiences of the world. As such, religion provides a powerful worldview and a specific epistemological and hermeneutical framework within which people seek to understand, interpret and make sense of themselves, their lives and their daily experiences in sickness and in health. Religions also have access to symbolic avenues of expression, such as rituals, prayers and worship, which can be used as powerful tools within the process of health development and care. While some theorists argue that religion can be detrimental to health (Ellis, 2000; Freud, 1968) there is also evidence to suggest that religion can be beneficial to the development and maintenance of health (Koenig *et al.*, 2001). As such, it is a form of spirituality that needs to be taken seriously.

The sacred

In a slightly different mode, but with clear resonance towards religion, the recent movement towards an emphasis on 'the sacred' is a helpful way to frame the tasks of spiritual care. Here spirituality is understood in terms of a more general sense of transcendence which may or may not include God but which certainly includes a sense of encountering something beyond the material norm and, indeed, of recognising the transcendent in the everydayness of life.

A significant proponent of this view is the American psychologist Kenneth Pargament. Pargament (2007) defines spirituality in terms of the sacred and the human propensity to sanctify objects, places, people and things. He argues that to sanctify something is to set it apart as somehow holy or sacred. Pargament uses the term 'sanctification' to refer to the process:

> ... *through which people view seemingly secular aspects of life as holding significance and character. Sanctification may be best understood as a different way of perceiving the world ... when people sanctify, they look at life through a sacred lens ... Through this lens, the visual field shifts and changes. What once appeared monochromatic, unidimensional, and ordinary becomes multicoloured, multilayered, mysterious, rich, unique, awesome, alive and powerful.*
>
> Pargament, 2007, p. 35

In this way the apparently mundane is transformed into transcendence through this process of sanctification. For some people, the process of sanctification relates to seeing the transcendent as being involved in apparently mundane aspects of daily life. Thus some people discover the transcendent within their families, their communities, their relationships with nature, and so forth. Again, 'people can also sanctify objects indirectly by attributing qualities to them that are associated with the divine' (Pargament, 2007 p.38), so objects, places and artefacts can all be imbued with divine significance. For example, a person with a crucifix beside their bed is doing much more than simply decorating their bedside! The crucifix is imbued with meaning; it may actually be a place where God physically is. Likewise people may sanctify other ordinary objects and things such as religious icons, the chapel or even pictures of loved ones. This process of sanctification occurs in many different places and many different forms. Carers need to be alert to the hidden spiritual meanings that practices and objects might have for their patients and the ways in which patients turn that which appears normal and everyday into something of divine importance.

Religion and the processes of sanctification that emerge from it thus remain an important aspect of spiritual care. Negatively, a focus on religion and transcendence can be considered anachronistic and irrelevant for at least two reasons. First, it is clear that there is massive decline in religion within Europe. It is not therefore immediately obvious why nurses should take religion as a significant aspect of their caring activities (Paley, 2008). If religion is no longer a cultural force, and if most of the patients that nurses will deal with will not be religious, why, it could be argued, would we spend time reflecting on such issues? Second, within a healthcare system that seeks to offer care that is generic and universally acceptable to 'all faiths and none', a focus on any particular traditions appears to be inappropriate and even offensive. The difficulty with the particularity of religion within a secular health service was highlighted recently by the case of an English nurse who was suspended simply for offering to pray with a patient (Alderson, 2009).

These two objections can be eased by realising two things. First, that there is evidence to suggest that the secularising thesis is not holding up to the empirical reality of the UK. It is true that *certain forms* of religion are dying out, however other forms of religion are increasing (Islam and evangelical Christianity, to name just two). There is also some evidence to suggest that people are not necessarily becoming less religious, rather they are becoming disillusioned with *formal* religious structures. The idea of 'ordinary religion', namely a religion that is much more personal and less dependent on formal structures, is one which is worth reflecting on. The idea that religion is an anachronism is simply wrong.

Second, to ignore the particular in preference to the universal is a bad policy for good healthcare practice. Kenneth Pargament (2002) has offered a useful critique of certain aspects of the 'religion and health' movement, particularly with assumptions that there is a monolithic 'thing' called 'religion' that can be measured and assumed to be good for one's health (we will look at this more fully below). He criticises the idea that religion has universal benefits. It is in the particularities of religion and religious practices that any meaningful health benefits are discovered. He makes five observations:

- the efficacy of religion varies by the kind of religion
- the efficacy of religion varies by the criteria of well-being

- the efficacy of religion varies by the person
- the efficacy of religion varies by context and situation
- the efficacy of religion varies by the degree religion is well integrated.

This brings to mind the crucial point that *spirituality may be universal but it is worked out in the particularities of people's lives*. Spirituality in its religious form requires that nurses come close to the person and really listen to what it is that they are saying. Religion is complicated and it is profoundly important in the way that it shapes people's experiences of illness. It is simply not enough to know that a person is a Muslim, a Christian, a Hindu, or a Jew. These 'banner headings' on their own tell us very little. It is only when we come close and listen to the personal intimate meanings of someone's religion that we can begin to offer anything like person-centred care. That being so, to argue that nurses should not develop such skills or that such skills are not important seems more than a little odd. In terms of spiritual assessment, this observation is vital.

Religion as projection

Another way in which religion enters the clinical sphere is through the mechanism of projection. This idea stems from the thinking of Freud (1968). Put simply it assumes that all religion is *nothing but* a projection of inner psychological needs and desires. It will be helpful to spend a little time thinking about the implications of this suggestion.

Freud perceived the mind in a quite particular way: as a hydraulic system. He imagined that within the mind there was a sea of psychic forces that is moving and constantly responding to the waves of psychic experience that human beings encounter throughout the life cycle. One of the primary desires of humans is to avoid anxiety. This being so the mind has various mechanisms that it uses to defend itself against anxiety and trauma. One could imagine it like this. A person experiences a psychic trauma of some sort. In order to avoid and deal with the anxiety that this event evokes, the person pushes (represses) the psychic event down into the psychic sea of the mind. However, because the mind is a hydraulic system, inevitably this disruption that is pushed down into the 'psychic sea' will cause an equivalent amount of psychic energy to pop up somewhere else (i.e. the symptom). However the thing that 'pops up' will be in a different form from the original trauma. The task of therapy is to trace back to the original trauma and to work on that psychic wound in order that the symptom can be overcome and equilibrium restored to the psychic sea.

According to Freud, much of the psychic disruption that people experience emerges from traumas and disappointments within childhood, primary amongst them the fact that one's father, whom one loves, adores and desires to care for you, to protect you and offer you safety at all times, will inevitably let you down. So, what happens? That trauma is pushed down into the psychic sea and emerges in a different form. In this case, our earthly father disappoints us and lets us down. So what do we do? We project our desires, hopes and expectations of our earthly father onto a transcendent screen: we create God the heavenly father in response to our disappointment with our earthly father. So in the end, religion turns out to be a form of mental illness! The task of the psychiatrist is to recognise religion as a pathological symptom and to do all that he or she can to help the person to get rid of it and return to a state of psychic equilibrium.

This of course is a simplistic version of Freud's complex theory, but I think it captures the essence for current purposes. The key point here is that religion and God are presumed not to be realities. They are psychic constructions, projections of human desires. As such they can't possibility be of any kind of therapeutic benefit. Implicitly and explicitly this perspective has been very influential, particularly within the area of mental health. Importantly, as John Hull (1996, p. 41) points out, adherence to positions such as Freud's (and Marx's) has created 'a lack of confidence in religious belief' and 'has been such that people today are suspicious of the spiritual. There is a cultural bias against religion so powerful that people are unable to accept their own religious and spiritual experiences.' This is no small point.

While Freud may have noticed something significant about the ways in which people construct ideas about God from human expectations and then project them onto God, his theory is questionable on two fronts. First, a good deal of his thinking is speculative and imaginative rather than empirical and proven. There is much that one might intuitively grasp onto within Freud's theory, but finding empirical evidence to support it is more difficult. This is somewhat ironic bearing in mind that a common criticism of belief in a God is that there is no empirical evidence to support such a claim. Freud's theory is inferential at best. That is, once one accepts the theory, one can infer various assumptions about human behaviour. But you have to first accept the theory, a theory that has no empirical basis. Freud and religion seem to be working on remarkably similar premises.

Second, and more substantially, if David Hay is correct about the relational nature of human beings and the social construction of secularism, then this is a significant challenge to the idea that religion is *nothing but* a psychic construction. The biological approach argues precisely the opposite of Freud's position. The strength of the biological approach at this point is that there is a reasonable evidence base to indicate that its premises may at least be plausible. It would therefore be unwise to take an uncritical approach to the idea that religion is simply a projection of human desires. It may in fact be secularism that is a projection of cultural desires.

Having said all of that, it is pretty clear that people do use projection when they are constructing their understandings of religion, and in particular their images of God. If you press religious people, it can become quite clear that their understanding of who God is and what God does is strangely similar to what they are and what they do … only bigger! For example, 'I am strong, God is stronger', 'I am loving, God is love', 'I protect my children, God protects us like His children'. Such projections may well stand in tension with established understandings from within the person's religious tradition. All this helps to reinforce the point made previously about not making assumptions about what a person believes or how they think about God simply by looking at which religious tradition they claim to adhere to. While Freud's position is deeply flawed, there remains something important that we can get from it if we reflect on it critically in the light of the other approaches we describe within this chapter.

Religion as behaviour

The third dimension of religion and religious spirituality relates to what has become known as the 'religion and health movement'. Here spirituality is understood as relating to the particular behaviours by which people practice their religion and engage in religious structures and the particular health benefits that they receive through such engagement. This approach has no real formal interest in whether or not any particular belief structure is 'true' or otherwise. Its focus is simply on what occurs when people operationalise (put into action) their religious beliefs and assumptions and the perceived and measurable health benefits that arise from such actions. It does not attempt to define what spirituality *is*. Rather it seeks to record, measure and assess what people who are spiritual (usually religious) *do* when they claim to be acting spiritually and the impact it has on their well-being. The focus of the religion and health perspective is on spiritual practices such as prayer, meditation, church attendance, religious affiliation, health-enhancing behaviours, social supports and enhanced psychological states (Chatters, 2000; Koenig, 1998; Koenig, Larson and McCullough, 2001). According to Larson, Swyers and McCullough (1997) and Swinton and Pattison (2001) spirituality has been associated with:

- extended life expectancy
- lower blood pressure
- lower rates of death from coronary artery disease
- reduction in myocardial infarction
- increased success in heart transplants
- reduced serum cholesterol levels
- reduced levels of pain in cancer sufferers
- reduced mortality among those who attend church and worship services
- increased longevity among the elderly
- reduced mortality after cardiac surgery.

People working with this approach do at times speak about the more general term 'spirituality,' However, it is clear that the majority of the research carried out so far focuses primarily on religion, and for the most part Christian religion.

This way of looking at religion is quite helpful in that it claims to provide an evidence base to support the use of religion in a healthcare context, thus providing an appropriate foundation for spiritual care at least in its religious mode. However, it has been pointed out that a good deal of the work done in this area is methodologically questionable (Sloane, 2006) and is based on the assumption that there is a unified, universal entity called 'religion' which can be measured using global scales. I have already indicated that this may not be the best way to look at religion and how religion functions in people's lives. Probably the most convincing research is that done on church communities (Gartner *et al.*, 1991). It seems apparent that adherents of religious communities have better health and are less likely to suffer from such things as depression and anxiety than those who do not belong to such communities. This is helpful, but it doesn't tell us as much as it claims to. It doesn't, for example, tell us anything about *why* people are attending churches or precisely *what* it is that they are getting from it. As Richard Sloane puts it: 'Anyone who believes that sitting in church makes you a Christian must also believe that sitting in a garage makes you a car!' (Sloane, 2006).

Without the knowledge gained from the type of perspective outlined by Pargament earlier in this chapter, the religion-as-behaviour model can actually obscure as much as it enlightens. Perhaps the most significant critique of this way of looking at religion and health emerges from the question: 'Should religion be viewed from a health perspective?' It is arguable whether the intention of most religious systems (with the possible exception of the Christian Scientist movement and the Seventh Day Adventists) is to focus on the attainment of health, at least not health as it is defined by the medical model. Indeed many religions call for sacrifices, which can be significantly detrimental to health. It would be an interesting exercise, for example, to go through the medical records of some of the church missionary organisations and look at the health experiences of the early missionaries. A religion that calls a person to up-stakes, leave home and go to a country where they are open to new and potentially deadly forms of viruses and infections may have been very bad for their health! The intention of most religions is to enable people to relate to God and this is a process that is not determined by the health effects of particular beliefs and practices. To reduce religion to its measurable manifestations seems a strange contradiction of a truly holistic approach.

The religion-as-behaviour perspective certainly has a place in our understanding and assessment of spirituality, but that place needs to be worked out in critical conversation with the other approaches I have outlined in this chapter.

Conclusion

In this chapter I have tried to provide a critical framework for approaches to spirituality that will lay a foundation for the various forms of assessment outlined in this book. I would stress that there is no single approach to spirituality and therefore to spiritual assessment. The nature of spirituality requires a plurality of approaches that recognise and respond to the complex nuances of that area of human experience that we have chosen to name 'the spiritual'. The framework presented here will, I hope, provide some foundational practical and theoretical marking points that will enable nurses and others to negotiate this complex terrain.

References

Ai, A. (2001). 'Integrating spirituality into professional education: A challenging but feasible task.' *Journal of Teaching in Social Work*, **22**(1/2), 103–30.

Alderson, A. *Telegraph*, 31 Jan 2009. Available at: http://www.telegraph.co.uk/health/healthnews/4409168/Nurse-suspended-for-offering-to-pray-for-patients-recovery.html (last accessed May 2010).

Barnum, B.S. (1996). *Spirituality in Nursing from Traditional to New Age*. New York: Springer.

Chatters, L.M. (2000). 'Religion and health: Public health research and practice.' *Annual Review of Public Health*, **21**, 335–67.

Cobb, M. and Robshaw, V. (1998). *The Spiritual Challenge of Health Care*. Oxford: Churchill Livingston.

Dawson, P.J. (1997). 'A reply to Goddard's "spirituality as integrative energy".' *Journal of Advanced Nursing*, **25**(2) 282–89.

Ellis, A. (2000). 'Can rational emotive behavior therapy (REBT) be effectively used with people who have devout beliefs in God and religion?' *Professional Psychology: Research and Practice*, **31**(1), 29–33.

Frankl, V. (1997) *Man's Search for Meaning*. Boston, MA: Beacon Press, pp. 122–29.

Freud, S. (1968). *The Future of an Illusion. The Standard Edition of the Complete Psychological Works of Sigmund Freud*. Volume 21. Translated by James Strachey. London: Hogarth Press.

Gartner, J., Larson, D.B. and Allen, G.D. (1991). 'Religious commitment and mental health: A review of the empirical literature.' *Journal of Psychology and Theology*, **19**, 6–25.

Hardy, A. (1965). *The Living Stream*. London: Collins.

Hay, D. (2006a). *The Spirit of the Child*. London: Jessica Kingsley Publishers.

Hay, D. (2006b). *Something There: The Biology of the Human Spirit*. London: Darton, Longman and Todd.

Hull, J. (1996). 'The ambiguity of spiritual value'. In: J.M. Halstead and M. Taylor (eds) *Values in Education and Education in Values*. London: Falmer Press, pp. 33–44.

Johnson, B., Tompkins, R. and Webb, D. (2002). *Objective Hope – Assessing the Effectiveness of Faith-Based Organizations: A Systematic Review of the Literature*. New York: Manhattan Institute for Policy Research, Center for Research on Religion and Urban Civil Society.

Kirsh, B. (1996). 'A narrative approach to addressing spirituality in occupational therapy: Exploring personal meaning and purpose'. *Canadian Journal of Occupational Therapy*, **63**, 55–61.

Kirsh, B., Dawson, D., Antolikova, S. and Reynolds, L. (2009). 'Developing awareness of spirituality in occupational therapy students: Are our curricula up to the task?' *Occupational Therapy International*, **8**(2), 119–25.

Koenig, H.G. (1998). *Handbook of Religion and Mental Health*. San Diego: Academic Press.

Koenig, H.G., Larson, D.B., and McCullough, M.E. (2001). *Handbook of Religion and Health*. New York: Oxford University Press.

Larson, D.B., Swyers, J.P. and McCullough, M. (1997). *Scientific research on spirituality and health: A consensus report*. Rockville, MD: National Institute for Healthcare Research.

Levin, J. (2001). *God, Faith, and Health: Exploring the Spirituality–Healing Connection*. New York: John Wiley and Sons.

Macmurray, J. (1961). *Persons in Relation*. London: Faber and Faber.

Markham, I. (1998). 'Spirituality and the world faiths.' In: M. Cobb and V. Robshaw (eds) *The Spiritual Challenge of Healthcare*. Oxford: Churchill Livingstone, pp. 73–89.

Newberg, A.B., d'Aquili, E.G. and Rause, V.P. (2001). *Why God Won't Go Away: Brain Science and the Biology of Belief*. New York: Ballantine Publishing.

Paley, J. (2008). 'Spirituality and nursing: A reductionist approach.' *Nursing Philosophy*, **9**(1) 3–18.

Pargament, K.I. (2002). 'The bitter and the sweet: An evaluation of the costs and benefits of religiousness.' *Psychological Inquiry*, **13**, 168–81.

Pargament, K.I. (2007). *Spiritually Integrated Psychotherapy: Understanding and Addressing the Sacred*. New York: Guilford Press.

Powell, A. (2001). 'Spirituality and science: A personal view.' *Advances in Psychiatric Treatment*, **7**: 319–21.

Powell, A. (2003). *Psychiatry and Spirituality – The Forgotten Dimension*. Washington: Pavilion/National Institute for Healthcare Research.

Reeves Roy, R. (2009). 'What is the role of spirituality in mental health treatment?' *Journal of Psychosocial Nursing and Mental Health Services*, **47**(3), 8–9.

Shelly, J.A. and Miller, A.B. (1999). *Called to Care: A Christian Theology of Nursing*. Downers Grove, IL: InterVarsity Press.

Sims, A. (1994). 'Psyche – spirit as well as mind?' *British Journal of Psychiatry*, **165**, 441–46.

Sloane, R. (2006). *Blind Faith: The Unholy Alliance of Religion and Medicine*. New York: St Martin's Press.

Swinton, J. (2001). *Spirituality and Mental Health Care: Re-Discovering a 'Forgotten' Dimension*. London: Jessica Kingsley.

Swinton, J. and Pattison, S. (2001). 'Come all ye faithful: Spirituality and healthcare practices.' *The Health Services Journal*, **111**, 24–25.

Swinton, J. and Mowat, H. (2006). *Practical Theology and Qualitative Research*. London: SCM Press.

Chapter 3
Recognising spiritual needs
Aru Narayanasamy

Introduction

As readers would have derived from the preceding chapters, a range of perspectives prevail about the nature of spirituality. One view is that if spirituality is elusive to definitions, then it is best not to dabble with it in clinical practice. The other contentious perspective is that spirituality is an invented notion, alluding to the point that there is no such thing as spirituality and therefore it is meaningless to both patients and clinical practice. In particular, Paley (2008) and Henery (2003) have generated an extensive critique of spirituality in nursing on the grounds that it is a reification that is uncritically accepted in healthcare practice. While these authors may have some justification in their discourses, to be dismissive of the spirituality of nursing in the light of their observation is misguided because extensive evidence amplifies its significance. Discarding the notion of spirituality based on this questionable stance is no solution. It is out of the question, since the genie is already out of the bottle.

The consensus and contradictions about spirituality in nursing and healthcare are given comprehensive attention in McSherry (2007). However, the stance taken in this chapter is that spirituality is the essence of our being and one that gives meaning and purpose to our very existence (Narayanasamy, 2006). To be dismissive of this need is tantamount to gross negligence of the very nature of the person. It matters because spirituality is a real and lived experience for many individuals. Indeed, Johnston Taylor (2007) calls for embedding of spirituality in everyday transaction and behaviour in clinical practice. The North American Nursing Diagnosis Association (NANDA) has accepted the dual diagnoses for spirituality: spiritual distress and readiness for enhanced spiritual well-being (Wilkinson, 2000). The subsequent sections in this chapter are based on the premise that the essence of our being needs attention in health and illness.

Holistic view

Holistic view

The holistic view draws our attention to spiritual needs. It is based on the premise that we all have needs and these are regarded as social, psychological, physical and spiritual. This is supported by Clark *et al.* (2003) who believe that a holistic view of healthcare is developing, where emotional and spiritual needs are considered inextricably from physical and psychological needs. Clarke *et al.* (2003) highlight the Joint Commission on Accreditation of Healthcare Organizations (JCAHO) as acknowledging that the psychosocial, spiritual and cultural values of patients have an effect on how they respond to their care. According to Wright (2005), looking at well-being and health should involve holism, which has its origins in words such as 'healthy', 'whole', 'holy'and 'hearty', as well as having connotations with healing.

Provision of spiritual care in response to spiritual needs should be given as readily as any other aspect of healthcare, regardless of the ailment. For example, Doherty (2006) provides a good demonstration of this by exploring the spiritual needs of patients and finding that individuals with dementia have spiritual needs that can be met regardless of how far their illness has progressed. According to Bell and Troxel (2001), there are a number of spiritual needs that patients may have. These include being connected, being respected, being appreciated, having the opportunity to love and be loved, being known and accepted, being compassionate, giving and sharing, and being productive and successful and hopeful.

In addition, Doherty (2006) highlights that patients experiencing a sense of loss may portray the following reactions in response to their illness: anger, anxiety, suspicion, sadness, hopelessness, worthlessness, grief, depression, despair, guilt, dismay, mourning of previous self, and acceptance that things will not be the same again. Doherty (2006) suggests that grief work and therapeutic interventions could be a good way of administering to these spiritual needs. She stresses that an adaptive approach is ideal, because individuals with different types of clinical problems react with different personalities to produce different circumstances. A tick-box approach to care would be unwise.

Spiritual needs

Scholars direct us to various categories of spiritual needs (Johnston Taylor, 2007). Bradshaw's (1972) taxonomy of needs may be used in clinical practice (Narayanasamy, 2001) to make sense of patients' spiritual needs. Powers (2006) develops a philosophical discourse on needs and argues that the concept of need is used in a variety of ways in nursing theory and practice. Powers argues that in nursing the concept of need is a top-down, mechanistic, means-to-an-end, product-oriented list of technical functions. However, this chapter addresses spiritual needs as a part of the holistic approach in which the patient is on the centre stage in the caring relationship.

Bradshaw (1972) identified four types of needs: normative, comparative, felt, and expressed.

Normative needs: These are those identified by professional experts and reflect those professionals' judgements and standards. Normative definitions of spiritual needs reflect professionals' views about the nature of health problems, which may vary from a lay person's perspective of their spiritual needs.

Comparative needs: Assessing comparative needs usually entails estimation by professionals of which group of patients is in greater need of spiritual care. Assessing needs in this way may bring into question how professionals judge which group needs what.

Felt needs: These are those that individuals themselves identify. Patients may reveal these if asked appropriate questions related to their spiritual needs. However, sometimes individuals may feel unable to disclose felt needs or some may not believe themselves to be 'in need'.

Expressed needs: These are what individuals say they need, and usually involve the turning of a felt need into a request or call for attention.

Maslow's hierarchy of needs

However, Maslow (1968) postulated a hierarchy of needs model in his humanistic theory of motivation. Maslow suggests that human needs can be placed along a hierarchy, where some will remain relatively unimportant until other needs have been fulfilled. The hierarchical nature of this model is well illustrated in Fig. 3.1 below.

Figure 3.1 **A hierarchy of needs**
based on Maslow (1968) and Narayanasamy (2001).

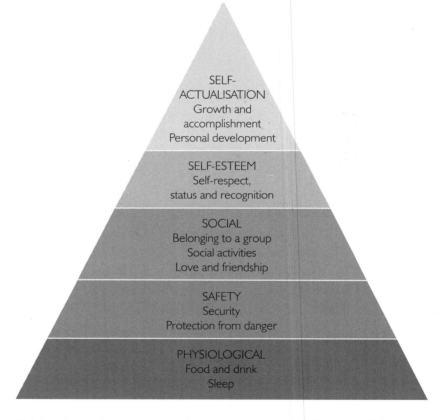

Spiritual needs can be explained in terms of Maslow's hierarchy of needs as outlined in the following case illustration from Narayanasamy:

> *Sylvia finds that her life has no longer meaning or purpose. She feels that life is drifting away and that she has not achieved anything significant although she previously had high ideals and aspirations. Sylvia told the practice nurse when*

receiving treatment that she is experiencing a great sense of despair and hopelessness. Sylvia disclosed to the nurse, 'I lack confidence and feel angry with others as they are always letting me down… Nobody values me for what I am. My family and friends try to take advantage of me and never appreciate what I do for them. The other day, as a favour I drove my friend to see her mother who lives miles away from her, and then on our way home she asked me to take her to the supermarket. After shopping I was looking forward to go home to have some time for myself, but she asked if I could collect her children from school as she had something important to do. She never returns a favour. I am fed up of people taking advantage of me. I feel angry with them but I can't bring myself to say no to them. I find my work boring and monotonous and nobody seems to care about me. I feel really fed-up and now this problem is making me worse. I've had enough.'

Narayanasamy, 2009, p. 3

Maslow's model explained

Apart from the basic physiological needs, humans use their senses to evoke certain feelings which are spiritual in nature, for example feeling peaceful and happy. They can use their senses of hearing (e.g. music) and smell (e.g. aromatherapy) to induce a sense of spiritual uplift. Moving on to the next needs – safety needs – individuals need to feel secure, and in this respect trusting relationships with others and their surroundings are considered to be spiritual needs (Sylvia feels insecure in her relationships) (Narayanasamy, 2006). On attainment of these needs, individuals are driven to experience a sense of belonging and love needs. It is well documented in the literature that humans become dispirited if these needs are not met (Sylvia feels that she is isolated and undervalued) (Narayanasamy, 2001). As part of our spirituality we need to feel a sense of belonging and being loved.

Next, our self-esteem needs are also important to our spiritual well-being. We need to feel a sense of achievement, worthiness, approval and recognition (Sylvia feels that her job is unfulfilling and unrewarding and that she is not being given any recognition by her friends). Any barriers to the achievement of these needs may cause us much spiritual distress and so these needs must be fulfilled before we move on to achieve self-actualisation, self-fulfilment and realisation of our own potential. It can be postulated that complete spiritual well-being equates with achievement of all needs as given in Maslow's hierarchical model of needs.

However, although Maslow offers a convenient way of explaining spiritual needs, his model can be problematic for two reasons when applying it in practice. First, needs placed in a hierarchy imply a degree of sophistication in distinguishing between needs in relative terms. In this respect, some needs appear more important than others, and some at the top of the hierarchy can be perceived to be more unattainable than others. The portrayal of needs in a hierarchy may imply a long struggle for some individuals to achieve self-actualisation. However, human experiences are not that clearcut and cannot be easily explained in terms of a model such as a hierarchy of needs. The second reason is that healthcare professionals experience difficulty in applying this model, even though it is popularly addressed in the literature. Factors such as stability, time, relationships, resources and so on act as barriers for professionals to promote spiritual well-being through conscious application of this model of needs. Powers (2006) is critical of Maslow's work (Maslow, 1968) as lacking a definition of needs and argues that in reality it is difficult to work through people's needs in as orderly way as is depicted in Maslow's heirarchy. However, it offers a useful framework for understanding spirituality as a human dimension.

We express our spiritual needs in a variety of ways and forms. Refer back to the case illustration of Sylvia on, pp. 40–41 and try to make a list of what her spiritual needs might be. You might identify some or all of the following:

- the need for meaning and purpose
- the need for love and harmonious relationships
- the need for forgiveness
- the need for a source of hope and strength
- the need for trust
- the need for expression of personal beliefs and values
- the need for spiritual practices, expression of concept of God or Deity and creativity.

Spiritual needs explored

**Spiritual
needs
explored**

Much of the discussion on spiritual needs that follows is largely derived from sources such as Narayanasamy (2001, 2006), McSherry (2007) and related evidence-based literature, as given in this section. Each of the spiritual needs is expanded as follows:

Meaning and purpose

During times of crisis, many of us find ourselves looking for meaning and purpose in our lives. This search for meaning and purpose may occur whether in illness or health. There is evidence to suggest that the search for meaning is a primary force in life in which we try to make sense of life in general as well as discovering meaning in suffering. You may come across patients who try to make sense of their affliction and the suffering that goes with it. The emphasis on meaning and purpose as central to our spirituality is depicted as a new 'postmodern' form of spirituality, as opposed to the historical or 'old' traditional form derived from religious and theocentric descriptors (McSherry, 2007).

There is evidence to suggest that patients struggle with finding a source of meaning and purpose in their lives (Peterson and Nelson, 1987; Rosseau, 2000). It is suggested that people with a sense of meaning and purpose survive more readily in very difficult circumstances and these include illness and suffering. Take, for example, Tom, who was a devout Christian with cancerous metastases to his bone, who defied the challenges of the crisis brought on by his illness and went on to live for many more years (Narayanasamy, 2006). I am sure that his faith provided meaning and purpose despite the devastating news about his cancer. There is some truth in the expression that he who has a 'why' to life can bear almost any 'how' (Frankl, 1967).

Rosseau's (2000) study into spirituality and the dying patient showed that with the approach of death, patients frequently begin an inward journey to consider the questions of human existence and the meanings of life and death. Rosseau (2000) suggests that every person who faces death desires to know that his or her life had a purpose and meaning; therefore physicians are obliged to provide support and assistance in addressing such spiritual concerns and in doing so to afford a peaceful death. Doherty (2006) adds that a lack of purpose can result in a sense of 'nothingness' and a decline in well-being and health.

Many of us approach the task of life in a variety of ways with varying degrees of ability to cope with a crisis. For some people, suffering may open–up the quest for new meaning and purpose. Narayanasamy (2006) postulates that there is a distinction between the religious and the apparently non-religious person in the way in which they approach spirituality. That is, the religious person experiences his or her existence not merely as a task but as a mission, and is aware of a taskmaster, the source of this mission. Religious scholars assert that source is God. There is evidence to suggest that some patients of faith claim that they derive further strength to cope with crisis.

For example, one patient claimed the following in another case studied by Narayanasamy:

> When they told me that I have cancer the news devastated me. I started to think about myself, my family and the future. I thought to myself what have I done to deserve this? It was terrible. I felt numb, confused, bewildered. Obviously, you feel terrible, who wouldn't in this situation. Then I started to think of the power above us… So I called for a Divine Power, in a way calling God to come and rescue me from this mess, if you like. You can say it is a sort of a belief in God to bail me out, really.
>
> Narayanasamy, 2006, p. 74

In a crisis such as bereavement the person going through it experiences meaninglessness, that is, he or she expresses a sense of bewilderment and loss of meaning. For example, people with a diagnosis of cancer, or at the end of life, or experiencing a major catastrophe all cry out for help in search of meaning, and desperately seek to talk to someone who will give attention and time to their exploration of meaning and purpose. Others may react by withdrawing and sinking into a state of meaninglessness, despair and hopelessness.

Some people who are searching for meaning and purpose may indicate a need for exploration of spiritual issues. In some instances the person in search of spirituality may want to talk about religious feelings – or lack of them. He or she may not be asking for advice or opinions, but simply for an opportunity to talk about feelings, to express doubts and anguish. Such opportunity for expression can bring about clarity and a renewed sense of meaning and purpose.

Those who have strong religious convictions and claim to sense the presence of their God may still need encouragement to adapt to unexpected changes. They are likely to experience hope even when their usual support systems let them down. Their felt experience of God reassures them that God will never fail them. In a meaning-making relationship, the nurse may have to act as a catalyst in helping the patient in crisis by establishing their relationship with God or a deity. Some patients may wish to pray as a way of maintaining their relationship with their God, and this may be tricky for nurses who are non-believers. Although the evidence so far is inconclusive, it is also indicative of a close association between prayer and healing (Narayanasamy and Narayanasamy, 2008). Prayer evokes the body–mind responses that promote healing in the broader sense. Apart from physical healing, prayer appears to promote the healing of emotions, inner feelings and relationships that may be more profound than physical healing.

Harold Koenig (1997) encourages healthcare practitioners to be involved in prayer for healing. Spiritual history or assessment of patients with acute and chronic illnesses should be part of the care intervention. It is paramount that nurses ascertain what role a patient's faith and prayer plays in helping them to cope (or whether it hinders it). It should be part of the routine when any spiritual needs are identified to refer the patient to the staff of a department of spiritual and pastoral care.

Love, harmonious relationships and connectedness

The need for love, harmonious relationships and connectedness are integral to meaning and purpose (McSherry, 2001; Narayanasamy, 2006; O'Brien, 2003). The need for love and to give love are fundamental human needs (Maslow, 1968). This is enduring throughout our lives. A spiritually distressed person requires unconditional love, that is love that has no strings attached to it. This is sometimes referred to as 'in spite of' love. The spiritually distressed person does not have to earn it by being good or attractive or wealthy. The person is simply loved for him or herself, regardless of faults or ignorance or bad habits or deeds.

Galek *et al.* (2005) also advocate the importance of love within spirituality. They found that patients desired not to be abandoned by their pastor, rabbi or spiritual advisor. They wanted to give and receive love and to experience the committed presence of others. According to Sherwood (2000), through the harmony of human to human connection, patients receive healing.

Deepak Chopra, the well-known writer about spirituality and health, epitomises love as central to our lives and, like Sherwood, highlights its healing properties. Using Eastern and Western dimensions of spirituality and medicine, Chopra makes substantive claims that love as a spiritual resource mends our brokenness to regain our wholeness as a person. He proposes that 'Love is spirit' and 'spirit is love' (p. 33) and consequently has devoted a whole book entitled *The Path to Love* to highlighting the spiritual significance of love (Chopra, 1997).

The notion of connectedness was mentioned before and is a common theme in the literature on spirituality. According to Rajakumar *et al.* (2008), when looking at spirituality and depression, spirituality was experienced as connections. For example, participants in his study spoke about making connection with God and a higher power. This connection had significant value because it enabled participants to start the process of accepting their depression and working towards recovery. Rajakumar *et al.* (2008) noted that such connections were made through prayer and, in some cases, this prevented the sufferers from committing suicide.

In addition to a connection with God, Rajakumar *et al.* (2008) found that recovery among the participants with depression was also aided by forming relationships with their spiritual self, with others, and with nature. The relationships functioned to reassure them that they were not alone in their struggles and not totally responsible for their depression. This realisation helped them to accept their life's struggles and also enabled them to move forward with their life. Connecting and relation-ships were associated with courage, creativity and a renewed sense of self. This is significant, because one characteristic symptom of depression is disconnection from one's environment.

The manifestations of the need for love are self-pity, depression, insecurity, isolation, and fear. These are indicators of a need for love from oneself, other people, and from God, if the person is religious. The person receiving this kind of love experiences feelings of self-worth, joy, security, belonging, hope and courage.

According to NANDA (Wilkinson, 2000), the following can be identified as signs of spiritual problems in a person who may need to receive love to resolve some of them:

- worries and expressions of concerns about how the rest of the family will manage after his or her death
- expression of feelings of a loss of faith in God
- reluctance to discuss feelings about dying with close friends and family
- failure to call on others for help when needed
- expression of fear of tests and diagnosis (although this is universal)
- expression of feeling lack of support from others
- behaviour that reflects he or she 'should' be conforming to the behaviour of a 'good' patient or person
- refusal to cooperate with the healthcare regimen
- expression of guilt feelings
- thoughts of confession and feelings about shameful events
- expression of anger with self or others
- expressions of ambivalent feelings toward God
- expression of despondency during illness or hospitalisation
- expression of resentment toward God
- expression of loss of self-value due to decreasing physical capacity
- expression of fear of God's anger
- desperate 'clinging' to those who talk to them.

As given in NANDA, spiritual distress is one of the many diagnoses (Wilkinson, 2000). The spiritually distressed person also has a need to give love, which may include, for example, worries about financial status of his or her family during hospitalisation or separation from their family and worries about separation from others by death.

Forgiveness

Writing from a psychological perspective, Professor Ann Macaskill (2002) provides an authoritative discourse on forgiveness which is central to spirituality. She implies that many individuals' lives are wrecked because of guilt feelings as well as the inability to forgive. In this regard, a state of dispiritedness may be a manifestation of guilt or the need to be forgiven.

Forgiveness can be seen from two sides: the need to both give and receive. A person who experiences spiritual distress expresses feelings of guilt and therefore requires the opportunity for forgiveness. The scenario described earlier depicts Sylvia's need to forgive herself, her friends and those responsible for her situation. Guilt often emerges when a person experiences the realisation that one has failed to live up to his or her own expectations or the expectations of others. For example, we may first experience guilt as a child when our behaviour does not measure up to the standards set for us by our parents. We contradict them and do the very things we are told not to do. Guilt breeds within us in the form of regrets, not only for the things we have done, but also for what we have not done. Unresolved conflicts in relationships can result in feelings of guilt, as depicted in this next scenario:

> *When I was talking to a patient he was filled with remorse about his wife's death. He attributed this to his careless driving when during one summer his car was involved in a road traffic accident and his wife died in the crash. He used our encounter as an opportunity to release his pent-up emotions and felt peaceful. My presence and willingness to listen instilled a sense of calm and perhaps a sense of release for the patient.*

Narayanasamy, 2006, p. 74

The feelings of guilt may be expressed as feelings of paranoia, hostility, worthlessness, defensiveness, withdrawal, or psychosomatic complaints, rationalisations, criticism of self or others or God, and 'scapegoating'. Evidence shows that forgiveness may bring about feelings of joy, peace and elation, and a sense of renewed self-worth (Macaskill, 2002; Narayanasamy, 2006; Steinhauser *et al.*, 2006).

Professor Ann Macaskill (2002) suggests that people who forgive almost always derive positive effects in terms of healing. The issue of forgiveness is closely linked with peace, as the former can bring about the latter. Forgiveness leads to resolution and this can be very comforting to the patient. According to Steinhauser *et al.* (2006), a recent qualitative study found that a positive end-of-life experience was associated with being at peace. Conceptual analysis found that for many respondents, the sense of peacefulness was related to the religious notion of being at peace with God. A sense of peacefulness may have resulted from a clear decision about whether to continue a course of chemotherapy or assurance that a patient's pain and symptoms would be managed.

The case of forgiveness is a clear example of how spirituality may involve religion, but it is not exclusively a mere synonym of religion. People who do not have a religion still have spiritual needs and may still desire peace and resolution. So how do these people achieve this? Steinhauser *et al.* (2006) suggests that it is still through the process of forgiveness, but it may include resolving a conflict with a family member or loved one, within themselves, or in a spiritual reflection on the meaning of illness in their lives. Steinhauser *et al.* (2006) add that resolution within the biomedical, psychosocial, or spiritual domains of patients' experiences often precedes the subjective experience of peacefulness.

Hope and strength

Galek *et al.* (2005) acknowledge the power of hope and gratitude to nourish patients and replenish their spirit. Hope has the capacity to connect with the possibilities of realities beyond the self. Many patients have the need to feel hopeful, to feel a sense of peace and contentment, to keep a positive outlook, to have a quiet space to meditate or reflect, to be thankful or grateful, and to experience laughter and humour. Ross (1997) found a link between hope and the will to live. For many of us our sense of hope can be a powerful motivator in enabling an open attitude toward new ways of coping (Herth and Cutcliffe, 2002). The spiritually distressed person may experience a feeling of hopelessness, and the hopeless person may see no way out; there may be no other possibilities other than the most dreaded – suicide.

We thrive on good relationships with others and this is another facet of our hope (Narayanasamy, 2006). This includes relationships with others, ourselves and the world, whether a person believes that what is desired is possible. In the scenario described earlier (pp. 40–41) Sylvia needs to form new relationships and perhaps take an interest in new leisure pursuits or change her job to give her new hope.

Hope is also necessary for future plans. Further sources of our hope include seeking support, love and the stability provided by important relationships in our life, and putting into action our future plans. If a patient believes in God, then hope in God is important. For believers, this hope in God is the ultimate source of strength and supersedes all aspirations that are transitional.

Hope is central to our need for a source of strength. We derive strength from our hope as it gives us the courage needed to face innumerable odds in a crisis. Religious people appear to draw strength from hope through prayer because of their relationship with God or a Supreme Being. The patients in Haase's study (1987) concurred that belief in the power of prayer helped them cope with medical procedures, and opportunities to express their faith helped them resolve the situation they found themselves in. For some, communication with God and prayer is a source of strength, and more recent studies suggest similar findings (Benson and Stark, 1996; Koenig, 2001; Narayanasamy, 2006.) Sylvia, in the case illustration, requires a message of hope that may provide energy, strength and courage for taking new directions in her life.

Trust

A sense of trust is paramount in most relationships. As humans, we feel secure when we can establish a trusting relationship with others. In the scenario, Sylvia appears to be spiritually distressed and is in need of a trusting relationship. Nurses and healthcare practitioners can create an environment which demonstrates that carers make themselves accessible to others, both physically and emotionally. Trusting is the ability to place confidence in the trustworthiness of others and this is essential for spiritual health and total well being (Narayanasamy, 2001, 2006). Learning to trust in an environment which is alien can be a daunting task and not an easy skill to accomplish. A trusting relationship and friendship, in the case of Sylvia and patients like her, may help to set them on track for spiritual wellness.

What follows is a scenario from an on-going research study by Narayanasamy that captures spiritual care in practice.

Adam, a staff nurse on a ward for palliative care, was able to respond to his patient's spiritual needs because of the rapport and trust that he built with his patients. Adam responded to a palliative care patient by recognising that he had very specific wishes with regard to his spirituality. He wanted to die in peace. Adam helped the patient to discuss his feelings about the need to complete some unfinished business such as to 'set his house in order'. He wanted candles to be lit before he died and finally he wanted his closest family and friends to be present at the end. Adam told me that the patient's relatives felt very pleased and satisfied with all the care they gave.

Narayanasamy, 2009, p. 12

Personal beliefs and values

The opportunity to express personal values and beliefs is a known spiritual need (Narayanasamy, 2006). In this sense, spirituality refers to anything that a person considers to be of highest value in life. Sylvia (p. 41) appears spiritually distressed because her state of mind is such that she is unable to find value in what she does. A supportive friendship may enable her to regain a sense of value in life. Personal values that may be highly regarded by an individual include, for example, beliefs of a formalised religious path; for others it may be a set of very personal philosophical statements, or perhaps a physical activity or new hobby.

Spiritual practices, concept of God or Deity and creativity

The opportunity to express our needs related to spiritual practices, the concept of God or Deity, and creativity may present as a feature of spirituality. The concept of God or Deity may be an important function in the inner life of a person. The need to carry out spiritual practices concerning God or Deity may be too daunting for the person if the opportunity is not available or the environment is alien or unreceptive to this need.

Spiritual care transcends cultural and religious differences and the following scenario (part of an on-going research study) captures this well:

In spite of the cultural and religious difference, staff nurse Helen describes how she responded to a patient's spiritual needs. She recounted that a patient of the Sikh faith was ventilated and treatment was to be withdrawn. The family was large and extended, they expressed certain wishes as to last offices, all were distraught and wailed and chanted. She had no idea what was expected of their rituals and religion. All she knew were that things had to be done differently, so she contacted the hospital chaplain to find out what was to be done in Sikh religion. She found a single room for the patient so that they had more privacy. She supported them as much as she could but at the same time gave them the space and privacy to grieve as the patient parted from them. Helen felt that the family were all very upset but grateful and very appreciative of her support and sensitivity to their spiritual needs.

Narayanasamy, 2009, p. 14

Our creative needs may feature in spirituality. A religious minister in a Connecticut Hospice uses the arts as an avenue to the spirit in which actors, writers, musicians and artists of a university are invited to exhibit their work and give performances (Wald, 1989). Galek *et al.* (2005) introduce the concept of 'The Divine', which they describe as the expression of spirituality through traditional religious rites and practices, which were identified as 'The Divine'. Many spiritual practices, rituals or services are designed to facilitate interconnection with the divine or sacred. Experiences of communion can help individuals realise their relationship with the transcendent. Practices leading to this experience can be diverse, from having someone to pray with you, or for you, performing rituals, attending services, or reading spiritual or religious materials.

Who should provide spiritual support?

Spiritual support

Opinions are divided about who should provide spiritual support based on spiritual assessment. My view is that at the least healthcare practitioners should be sensitive to the spiritual needs of their patients as there is sufficient empirical evidence to suggest that spiritual distress arises as a consequence of critical junctures, such as illnesses, in people's lives. However, only those who have undertaken additional professional development in the rudiments of spiritual care should provide spiritual support. Spiritual support based on effective spiritual assessment is a highly skilful activity (Narayanasamy, 2007). It requires education and experience in spiritual support. Sufficient information on spiritual needs is provided here to guide readers who are likely to give direct spiritual support, although indirect support may entail enlisting the help of a competent practitioner who is skilful in spiritual assessment and spiritual support. There is sufficient material here to give confidence to students and practitioners to be sensitive to their patients' spiritual needs. It is imperative that caring teams observe the following during healthcare interventions, including sensitivity to patients' spiritual needs:

- do not impose personal beliefs (or lack of them) on the patient or families
- respond to the patient's expression of need with a correct understanding of their background
- be sensitive to the patient's signals for spiritual and psychological support.

If a member of the caring team feels unable to respond to a particular situation of spiritual need, then they should enlist the services of an appropriately qualified member of staff or spiritual care team.

Healthcare interventions should be based on an action, which reflects caring for the individual. There is no cure without caring. Caring signifies to the person that he or she is significant, and is worth someone taking the trouble to be concerned about them. Caring requires actions of support and assistance in growing. It means adopting a non-judgemental approach and showing sensitivity to the person's cultural values, physical preference and social needs. It demands an attitude of helping, sharing, nurturing and loving.

Conclusion

Spiritual needs are identified and described in the light of the evidence that these are lived experience for many people whether in health or illness. The holistic perspective is used to justify the rationale for this chapter, although competing theories about the nature of spirituality and spiritual needs are emerging. In this chapter spiritual needs are explicated as: the need for meaning and purpose; the need for love and harmonious relationship; the need for forgiveness; the need for a source of hope and strength; the need for trust; the need for expression of personal beliefs and values; and the need for spiritual practice, expression of concept of God or Deity and creativity.

Spiritual needs are charted in a linear and logical fashion in order to capture and construct experiences as manifestations of spirituality to direct spiritual support for patients. In order to carry out spiritual assessment, the main theme of this book, it is imperative that this is underpinned by a sound understanding of what constitutes spiritual needs. The spiritual *needs* described in this chapter are by no means exclusive, but are increasingly recognised within the province of healthcare in the contemporary evidence on spirituality. It is imperative that the essence of the person is addressed. This requires nurses and health carers to be part of the journey in suffering as individuals try to make sense of their dispiritedness when challenged by health crises in their lives. Reaching out to those who require assistance, as they navigate and negotiate through rough and difficult terrains in their journey to recovery, is one of the greatest gifts one could offer.

References

Benson, H. and Stark, M. (1996). *Timeless Healing. The Power of Biology of Belief*. London: Simon and Schuster.

Bell, V. and Troxel, D. (2001). Spirituality and the person with dementia – A view from the field. *Alzheimers's Care Quarterly*, 2(2), 31–45.

Bradshaw, J. (1972). 'The concept of social need'. *New Society*, 19(3), 640–43.

Chopra, D. (1997). *The Path to Love*. London, Rider.

Clark, P.A., Drain, M. and Malone, M.P. (2003). 'Addressing patients' emotional and spiritual needs'. *Joint Commission Journal on Quality and Safety*. 29(12), 659–70.

Doherty, D. (2006). Spirituality and dementia. *Spirituality and Health International*, 7, 203–10.

Frankl, V.E. (1967). *Man's Search for Meaning*. New York: Washington Square.

Galek, K., Flannelly, K.J., Vane, A. and Galek, R.M. (2005). 'Assessing a patient's spiritual needs – A comprehensive instrument'. *Holistic Nursing Practice*, 19(2), 62–69.

Haase, J.E. (1987). 'Components of courage in chronically ill adolescence: A phenomenological study'. *Advances in Nursing Science*, 9(2), 64–80.

Henery, N. (2003). 'Constructions of spirituality in contemporary nursing theory'. *Journal of Advanced Nursing*, 42(6), 550–57.

Herth, K. and Cutcliffe, J.R. (2002). 'The concept of hope in nursing. 3: Hope and palliative care'. *British Journal of Nursing*, 11(14), 977–83.

Johnston Taylor, E. (2007). *What Do I Say? Talking with Patients about Spirituality*. Philadelphia, PA: Templeton Foundation Press.

Koenig, H.G. (1997). *Is Religion Good for Your Health?* New York: The Haworth Pastoral Press.

Koenig, H.G. (2001). *Spirituality in Patient Care: Why, How, When and What?* Radnor, PA: Templeton Foundation.

Macaskill, A. (2002). *Heal the Hurt: How to Forgive and Move On*. London: Sheldon Press.

Maslow, A.R. (1968). *Toward a Psychology of Being*. New York: Van Nostrand.

McSherry, W. (2001). 'Spiritual crisis? Call a nurse', in H. Orchard (ed.) *Spirituality in Health Care Contexts*. London: Jessica Kingsley.

McSherry, W. (2007). *The Meaning of Spirituality and Spiritual Care within Nursing and Health Care Practice*. London: Quay Books.

Narayanasamy, A. (2001). *Spiritual Care: A Practical Guide for Nurses and Healthcare Practitioners*. London: Quay Books.

Narayanasamy, A. (2006). *Spiritual Care and Transcultural Care Research*. London, Quay Books.

Narayanasamy, A. (2007). 'Palliative care and spirituality'. *Indian Journal of Palliative Care*, **13**(2), 32–41.

Narayanasamy, A. (2009). *Spirituality E-Learning Resource*. Nottingham: University of Nottingham.

Narayanasamy, A. and Narayanasamy, M. (2008). 'The healing power of prayer and its implications for nursing'. *British Journal of Nursing*, **17**(6), 394–404.

O'Brien, M.E. (2003). *Prayer in Nursing*. Boston: Jones and Bartlett.

Paley, M. (2008). 'Spirituality and nursing: A reductionist approach'. *Nursing Philosophy*, **9**, 3–8.

Peterson, E. and Nelson, K. (1987). 'How to meet your clients' spiritual needs'. *Journal of Psychosocial Nursing*, **25**(5), 34–38.

Powers, P. (2006). 'The concept of need in nursing theory'. In: H.S. Kim and I. Kollak (eds) *Nursing Theories: Conceptual and Philosophical Foundations*. New York: Springer.

Rajakumar, S., Jillings, C., Osborne, M. and Tognazzini, P. (2008). 'Spirituality and depression: The role of spirituality in the process of recovering from depression'. *Spirituality and Health International*, **9**, 90–101.

Ross, L.A. (1997). *Nurses' Perceptions of Spiritual Care*. Aldershot: Avebury.

Rosseau, P. (2000). 'Spirituality and the dying patient'. *Journal of Clinical Oncology*, **18**(9), 2000–02.

Sherwood, G. (2000). 'The power of nurse–client encounters'. *Journal of Holistic Nursing*, **18**(2): 159–75.

Steinhauser, K.E., Voils, C.I., Clipp, E.C., Bosworth, H.B., Christakis, N.A. and Tulsky, J.A. (2006). 'Are you at peace? One item to probe spiritual concerns at the end of life'. *Archive of Internal Medicine*, **166**, 101–05.

Wald, F.S. (1989). 'The widening scope of spiritual care'. *American Journal of Hospice Care*, **6**(4), 40–43.

Wilkinson, J.M. (2000). *Nursing Diagnosis Handbook with NIC Interventions and NOC Outcomes*, 7th edn. New Jersey: Prentice Hall.

Wright, S.G. (2005). *Reflections on Spirituality and Health*. London: Whurr.

Chapter 4
Spiritual assessment: definition, categorisation and features
Wilfred McSherry

Introduction

The subject of spiritual assessment in healthcare practice raises a number of conceptual, practical, organisational and ethical challenges. These challenges undoubtedly influence the nature and manner in which spiritual assessment is perceived, approached and undertaken. It also raises a number of questions about quality and governance and providing evidence for this aspect of care. Therefore, this chapter will explore what is meant by the idiom 'spiritual assessment'. The chapter will briefly introduce readers to the main classification of assessment tools currently documented in healthcare literature, in preparation for the deeper exploration that follows in subsequent chapters. It will also describe and discuss some of the factors and features influencing the implementation and success of spiritual assessment tools used within diverse healthcare contexts.

Context within healthcare

Context within healthcare

Up until recently, spiritual assessment was one of the most ignored aspects of assessment (Stoter, 1995). It was not really discussed or explored within healthcare literature. If one traces the antecedents of spiritual assessment tools, it seems that the idea of spiritual assessment was initially proposed and advanced by the nursing profession. More recently, models of spiritual assessment have been developed by other professions, for example within the field of social work (Hodge, 2001, 2005a, 2005b, 2006), medicine (Koenig, 2002; Puchalski and Romer, 2000) and mental health (Gilbert,

2008). Authors have also explored the implication of spiritual assessment for healthcare contexts and provided useful summaries and commentaries about the nature and technical implications of using such models. Examples include the work of Carson (1989), Cobb (1998), Swinton (2001), Taylor (2002), Robinson, Kendrick and Brown (2003), McSherry (2006) and Greenstreet (2006).

Stoll's guidelines

Stoll's guidelines

Ruth Stoll's pioneering *Guidelines for Spiritual Assessment* (Stoll, 1979) are probably the earliest attempt at offering some structure and guidance for conducting a comprehensive spiritual assessment within nursing practice. It would appear that these guidelines have provided a platform or a template around which spiritual assessment tools have evolved within a healthcare context.

Stoll (1979) presents a 'direct method' of spiritual assessment, outlining four primary areas (see Box 4.1).

Box 4.1

A 'direct method' of spiritual assessment in four primary areas (adapted from Stoll, 1979)

> **1. Concept of God or deity:** This examines theistic elements as well as religious elements.
>> Good questions to ask are:
>>> – Is religion or God significant to you?
>>> – Is prayer helpful to you?
>>> – What happens when you pray?
>
> **2. Sources of hope and strength:** These relate to sources of support, particularly surrounding people and relationships.
>> Good questions to ask are:
>>> – Who is the most important person to you?
>>> – To whom do you turn when you need help?
>
> **3. Religious practices:** these address the impact that an illness might have on the patient's ability to maintain religious practices.
>> Good questions to ask are:
>>> – Do you feel that your faith (religion) is helpful to you?
>>> – Are there any religious practices that are important to you?
>
> **4. Relationship between spiritual beliefs and health:** This explores existential issues about the patient's concerns or visions for the future.
>> Good questions to ask are:
>>> – What has bothered you most about being sick or about what is happening to you?
>>> – What do you think is going to happen to you?

A review of these four primary areas suggests that Stoll's model (Stoll, 1979) may not be appropriate for use in all healthcare contexts. At first glance, some of these questions appear intrusive and intimidating. Furthermore, the focus seems to be on religion and only apply to those individuals with a religious belief and faith. However, one needs to explore the historical context in which Stoll's work was undertaken. Her work is advisory and not an edict. She indicates that there is a need for flexibility and adaptability when using the guidance and emphasises that the assessment should always be led by the patient. Her work was developed within the USA where attitudes towards religious belief and practice are different from those in other parts of the world such as the UK. Therefore, the idea that such a model can be transferred and used without any adaptation or modification within other regions of the world is questionable. Stoll probably did not have this in mind as she was developing guidance for use in the USA. McSherry and Ross (2002) indicate that such direct methods of spiritual assessment may not be suitable to some areas of healthcare practice, particularly within acute and critical care. Despite these criticisms, Stoll's work has made a significant contribution to the development of spiritual assessment tools, offering a simple framework that enables nurses to engage with patients' spiritual needs. Adaptations of Stoll's original work can still be found in use within healthcare practice.

A noticeable absence of definition

Absence of definition

Following the publication of Stoll's seminal work, a great deal of literature and subsequent discussion has been devoted to the area of spiritual assessment. Despite all this activity, a noticeable omission is the lack of any real attempt to actually define what is meant by 'spiritual assessment'. A number of synonyms seem to be used when describing this phenomenon; for example, Maugens (1996) presents the idea of spiritual history, while McSherry (2007) speaks of spiritual narrative. Others introduce spiritual assessment in more generic terms: Highfield and Cason (1983) explore nurses' ability to recognise spiritual needs; Muncy (1996) makes reference to 'comprehensive spiritual assessment'; while Ledger (2005) speaks about the duty of nurses to meet patients' spiritual needs. Other authors have developed what I have termed acronym-based models that raise the awareness of spiritual issues during the patient consultation (Anandarajah and Hight, 2001; Govier, 2000; Highfield, 1993; Narayanasamy, 1999, 2001; Puchalski and Romer, 2000). More recently there is a noticeable shift from a generic discussion of spiritual assessment towards practical application for specific groups or contexts (Tanyi, 2006; Timmins and Kelly, 2008).

Many authors writing about spiritual assessment (myself included) make a major assumption that everyone fully understands what this idiom means. I use the word idiom because 'spiritual assessment' is a phrase that has been used in the healthcare literature without any real attempt to clarify or outline its properties or constituent parts. That is not to say people have not offered fleeting insights. Anandarajah and Hight (2001, p. 84), for example, describe spiritual assessment as 'the process by which healthcare providers can identify a patient's spiritual needs pertaining to care'. This is quite a broad statement highlighting my concern about the lack of clarity and definition. Pierce offers a definition of spiritual assessment as 'the process by which healthcare providers can identify a patient's spiritual needs pertaining to medical care' (Pierce, 2004, p. 39). It is interesting that these authors use the word 'process', supporting my belief that spiritual assessment necessitates engagement with a range of conceptual, organisational, practical and ethical issues.

My reasons for drawing attention to these debates are to highlight that:

- Individuals may have diverse perceptions and understandings of what constitutes a spiritual assessment.

- Spiritual assessment comes in many different formats and guises on the assessment spectrum.

I am not suggesting that an authoritative definition is required. On the contrary, I don't think this is plausible or achievable. Nevertheless, I feel that there is a need to have some fundamental principles or guidelines as to what constitutes spiritual assessment in order to build a foundation for further exploration of the conceptual, organisational, practical and ethical challenges that spiritual assessment undoubtedly raises within healthcare practice. The current literature on spirituality in healthcare informs us that there is a need to engage critically with the concept of spirituality so that it reflects the views of wider society and, more importantly, the evidence on which it is based includes sound philosophical and scientific reasoning (Clarke, 2009; Paley, 2008, 2009). Hodge (2001) offers a potential solution to some of these questions, suggesting integrating the narrative (qualitative) and interpretive (scientific) aspects associated with spiritual assessment. If we are to achieve this then there needs to be some delineation of the idiom 'spiritual assessment' and a brief classification of the different types of assessment tool.

A definition of spiritual assessment

A definition of spiritual assessment

In the absence of any definitive or authoritative definition of spiritual assessment I would like to offer some thoughts derived from several years spent researching, teaching and applying this concept within clinical practice. My understanding of spiritual assessment is that it is an attempt to *enquire* positively and unobtrusively with a patient/client or his or her carer into areas of life that are associated with their health and well-being. It is more than just an enquiry into physical health. It is an exploration of the person's psychosocial and spiritual functioning. For some people this enquiry will have its genesis in a religious belief, while for others it may be concerned with more general aspects of their humanity and about finding meaning and purpose in their current situation. This type of enquiry may be undertaken formally as part of an admission process or informally as the patient/client expresses a need. These assessments may be practitioner-led or patient/client-led (McSherry, 2007).

For me, this form of enquiry concerns the interaction of one human being with another within a caring relationship and therapeutic environment. The process may be undertaken verbally or in a written format. Essentially it requires that the healthcare professional deals with all patients/clients as individuals, responding in a sensitive, open and confident manner. Healthcare professionals must be aware of their own personal beliefs and values and the limitations of their own professional practice and expertise. This is certainly evident in the

Nursing and Midwifery Council's (2007) documentation on skills clusters for pre-registration, which describes how nursing care should be provided in a warm, sensitive and compassionate way, showing kindness and empathy.

Primarily, healthcare practitioners must safeguard and protect the interest of the patient/client at all times. Therefore, the undertaking of any spiritual assessment requires practitioners to be competent and possess self-awareness regarding their own understanding of the spiritual dimension (Greenstreet, 2006). This raises the idea of competence in spiritual care, which is receiving attention in the healthcare literature (Gordon and Mitchell, 2004; van Leeuwen *et al.*, 2009).

Spiritual assessment is not about imposing a set of rigid questions on an individual. It is about interaction and dialogue between the patient and the healthcare practitioner. This dialogue should always be initiated and guided by the patient, although on admission to any healthcare setting there should always be some formal enquiring into a person's religious and non-religious belief and practices so that this can be documented, and with the patient's consent the relevant referrals and support obtained. I feel this constitutes good practice and is promoting patients' and clients' human rights (Human Rights Act 1998) with regards to freedom to maintain religious practice.

A cautionary word

A cautionary word

My concern with spiritual assessment *per se* is the potential for it to fragment care and perpetuate a tick-box reductionist mentality. As indicated in this chapter, spiritual assessment may take on many forms or guises. Depending upon what format is used, how it is introduced and managed could result in spiritual assessment serving just another bureaucratic function with no value for the patient or client. Furthermore, spiritual assessment is not just a one-off exercise but should be something continuous in nature. Patients' and clients' needs are dynamic and their circumstances change – sometimes suddenly and dramatically. Therefore, spiritual assessment in whatever form must be responsive and sensitive to such changes. The National Institute for Health and Clinical Excellence recognises the need for responsiveness:

Teams should ensure accurate and timely evaluation of spiritual issues facilitated through a form of assessment based on recognition that spiritual needs are likely to change with time and circumstances. Assessment of spiritual needs does not have to be structured, but should include core elements such as exploring how people make sense of what happens to them, what sources of strength they can draw upon, and whether these are felt to be helpful to them at this point in their life.

National Institute for Health and Clinical Excellence 2004, p. 98

A spectrum of approaches and meanings

A spectrum of approaches

The literature suggests spiritual assessment is a broad inclusive phrase that can be mapped onto a spectrum of approaches (Fig. 4.1) ranging from a straightforward enquiry about someone's religious beliefs to conducting an in-depth spiritual history (Highfield and Cason, 1985; Taylor, 2002).

Figure 4.1 **Spectrum of approaches to spiritual assessment**

Enquiry into religious belief

In-depth spiritual history

Along this spectrum, practitioners may utilise or draw upon a range of techniques, instruments, scales, models and skills to aid them with the conducting of the assessment – although it is my suspicion that the general public do not share the same understanding as healthcare professionals! I tested this out by asking my wife about her understanding of the term 'spiritual assessment' and her reply was interesting:

'A questionnaire identifying what my spiritual beliefs are and for me personally it would have to address my religious belief.'

This simple illustration highlights the difficulty of using the phrase 'spiritual assessment'. It can conjure up a range of images and interventions concerning what people believe it to entail. I also recall admitting patients onto a medical ward with a nursing assessment tool based on Roper, Logan and Tierney's (1990) Activities of Daily Living model. One of the areas to be assessed was termed 'spiritual needs'. I used to ask the patients what this meant for them and their responses were predictable – 'C of E but I'm not practising' or 'I don't have a religion'. Suffice to say the box was removed when the documentation was revised several years later.

Approaches to spiritual assessment

Approaches to spiritual assessment

As outlined above, spiritual assessment can take many forms, ranging from a 'simple' enquiry about a person's religious affiliation and status to an in-depth exploration of a person's life and narrative. Burkhardt and Nagai-Jacobson (1985) and McSherry and Ross (2002, p. 486) recommend a two-tiered approach to spiritual assessment that may involve the following stages:

● A descriptive religious enquiry (for example, in some acute settings, initial assessment focuses only upon identifying the individual's religious beliefs, affiliations and practices).

● An in-depth assessment may follow for patients/clients whom the healthcare professional feels are displaying possible indicators of spiritual distress.

McSherry and Ross (2002) present a broad categorisation and summary of the main types of spiritual assessment tools documented within the healthcare literature (see Box 4.2).

Danger of assumptions

Danger of assumptions

For many healthcare professionals who are perhaps familiar with the language and nature of spirituality, spiritual assessment will be an extension of their professional role and practice. This is evident in Chapter 1 which outlined the drivers and professional agendas that have led to healthcare professionals undertaking spiritual

Box 4.2 **Categories of approach to a spiritual assessment**
(McSherry and Ross, 2002)

Direct method: Ask direct questions (see Box 4.1) about the patient's religious or spiritual beliefs to elicit information about his or her potential spiritual needs.

Indicator-based models: This reflects the spiritual diagnosis–spiritual distress approach to spirituality (Carpenito, 1983, p. 451) which identifies certain characteristics that may indicate underlying spiritual distress (e.g. expression of concern or anger, resentment and fear about the meaning of life, suffering, and death).

Audit tools: There are increasing attempts to assess the effectiveness of practitioners in providing spiritual care, and many institutions are setting their own standards, actively monitoring and auditing areas of religious and spiritual needs to establish how well they have been addressed.

Value clarification: Likert-type scales reveal the extent to which patients agree or disagree with a particular statement. Tools using these scales are quick to administer, and provide quantifiable measures for researchers. They also give useful insights into their own values and perceptions of the concepts being investigated.

Indirect methods: Observational methods gather information from various sources to establish the presence of spiritual needs. Consensus must be reached about who does the observing, what signs are looked for and how they are interpreted, and whether (and how) they are documented.

Acronym-based models: PLAN (Highfield, 1993), FICA (Puchalski and Romer, 2000) and HOPE (Anandarajah and Hight, 2001) all focus attention on specific areas associated with spirituality or spiritual care. They are all quick and flexible and can be incorporated into the general assessment process.

---

assessments. My work illustrates that when the term 'spirituality' is used within a public context or with patients then the phrase may take on different meanings (McSherry, 2004; McSherry and Cash, 2004). Thus healthcare must prevent the perpetuation of a purely professional discourse that seems to make assumptions and have a false expectation about what patients need in this area. The development of spiritual assessment must, therefore, reflect and incorporate the voice and understanding of the public (McSherry, 2004). This is especially important in today's culturally and religiously diverse society.

Fundamental steps

Fundamental steps

Closer inspection of the spectrum of approaches and the types of tool available reveals that spiritual assessment is not as straightforward as it first sounds. It is a complex process that requires careful preparation and planning. Irrespective of the approach adopted by a ward, organisation or institution, there are a number of fundamental steps that must be addressed both implicitly and explicitly by patients, practitioners and the organisation itself if spiritual assessment is to have any relevance or meaning (Box 4.3). If these steps are not considered and engaged with in a thoughtful and meaningful way, then any attempt to implement spiritual assessment will be unsuccessful. These steps suggest that spiritual assessment is a relational process, in that it is very much dependent upon the way that people and organisations relate and work together for the benefit of care (Rumbold, 2002).

Box 4.3

Fundamental steps for the inclusion of spiritual assessment

Conceptual: Addresses the way in which people define, perceive and understand the nature of spirituality.

Organisational: Acknowledges the importance of people, places and processes when undertaking a spiritual assessment.

Practical: Covers the practical implications when any form of spiritual assessment is introduced.

Ethical: Considers any ethical issues and potential dilemmas encountered with any type of spiritual assessment.

Conceptual difficulties and challenges

Conceptual difficulties

This section explores some of the conceptual difficulties associated with defining spirituality and how these have a bearing on the development of spiritual assessment tools. The literature on spirituality indicates that it is a multifaceted and multidimensional phenomenon. People's understanding may be dependent upon their own worldview and personal philosophy of the world. Therefore culture, religion, race, ethnicity and other social factors must be considered when constructing any form of spiritual assessment tool, since these factors have a significant influence on a person's conceptualisation of spirituality. Having stated this, there may be some commonalities that individuals may share in terms of understanding; for example, many people will speak about what gives their life meaning and purpose or who their main sources of support are.

Continuum of beliefs

Spiritual assessment concerns an enquiry into a continuum of beliefs, which generates conceptual dilemmas when defining and trying to assess and engage with people's spiritual needs. McSherry and Cash (2004, p. 155) refer to the 'cocktail nature' of spirituality because it is associated with a number of meanings. They argue that there is not one single common denominator that gives the word a precise meaning. These conceptual issues must be considered when developing any form of spiritual assessment tool, as any tool created must be inclusive so it can embrace and allow those who use it to engage with the wide range of meanings given to the term 'spirituality'.

A taxonomy of spirituality therefore must include many variants. Depending on a person's beliefs, values and life experiences, 'spirituality' can be applied to general theistic beliefs in a supreme being or deity, to specific religious beliefs and practices, or to more general concepts such as 'inner strength' or 'inner peace'. Views of spirituality can also be influenced by political and social ideologies. Phenomenological and existential approaches emphasise the intrinsic meaningfulness of lived experience itself. Spirituality can also be used to refer to mystical ideas of transcendence, including notions of life after death. These varied interpretations of spirituality share an implicit, if not explicit, assumption that it will affect the quality of someone's life

This is not an exhaustive taxonomy as there may be an infinite range of applications of the word. This range can however be seen as falling under two basic forms, an 'old' form, focusing on religious and theistic dimensions, and a 'postmodern' one, focusing on phenomenological and existential dimensions.

More critique?

Clarke makes the following suggestion:

The model currently on offer has been fuelled by unconscious irrational anxieties about proselytisation; anxieties that nurses will not be able to distinguish religion from spirituality; anxieties about nursing being associated with theology; and anxieties about nursing having shared knowledge. These anxieties have fuelled the drive towards existential and inclusive definitions of spirituality.

Clarke, 2009, p. 1672

I agree with Clarke (2009) that the concept of spirituality, especially within nursing, has lacked critique. Her perspective and criticism are welcome in that they will assist all involved in the development of spiritual assessment tools to reflect constructively upon the motives and approach being adopted in the delivery of spiritual care. I feel that the 'taxonomy of spirituality' – while being inclusive and perhaps existentially focused – offers a framework for providing individualised and person-centred care. I say this because the taxonomy demonstrates that individuals construct their own unique spiritualities and these views may change across the lifespan.

Spiritual assessment and mental capacity

One other conceptual issue that I would like to raise is the notion of intellect and rationality as prerequisites for spirituality. Many definitions of spirituality allude to the fact that a person's spirituality is dependent upon intellect that is dynamic, responsive and relational, and changes through introspection, experience and interaction with the world, with people and perhaps with their relationship with God or a higher power. This position takes on a different poignancy if one looks at it within the context of an ageing population in which the numbers of cases of dementia are expected to dramatically increase. I make reference to dementia since such individuals lose their intellectual capacity as the disease progresses. More conceptual debate must be devoted to these questions because the danger is that we perpetuate a model of spirituality that discriminates against many people within society. Therefore, the language of spirituality and future debates must engage with these conceptual challenges.

Organisational aspects

This step refers to the organisational context in which spiritual assessment tools are constructed. Careful attention must be given to the people, place and process before any spiritual assessment tool is constructed and used.

People: The patients'/clients' needs must be considered and the practitioners who will be using the tool must be consulted and involved in its construction and implementation.

Place: The healthcare setting and context are of vital importance and must guide the decision with regard to the type and nature of any tool.

Process: This relates to the operational use and ongoing evaluation of the tool.

It is my firm belief that there is no such thing as a 'generic' spiritual assessment tool. The success of any spiritual assessment tool is especially dependent upon the context in which it is to be used. A tool developed for use within a hospice or palliative care setting will be different to one used by a physician seeing a patient in an outpatient clinic, or a patient visiting a day surgery unit. Of paramount importance is the fact that the tool should focus upon the needs of the individual rather than on routine or procedure or achieving corporate strategies or national targets. Governance is crucial to the development and ongoing monitoring of the efficiency and effectiveness of spiritual care. Clear mechanisms and line of governance will ensure accountability and lead to better-quality outcomes. They will also ensure that tools are developed as appropriate for the specific patient/client group and the particular healthcare context. The National Institute for Health and Clinical Excellence (2004, p. 96) endorses what has been discussed:

> *It follows that spiritual care should not be viewed solely in terms of the facilitation of appropriate ritual, which has implications for the assessment of spiritual needs. The nature of support needed can range from an informal sharing of ideas about the ultimate purpose of existence to the provision of a formalised religious ritual. The appropriate means of meeting*

need will vary by location, resources and skills available and the nature of needs assessed.

National Institute for Health and Clinical Excellence, 2004, p. 96

Hunt, Cobb, Keeley and Ahmedzia (2003) describe how they established an audit group with multiprofessional representation and public involvement to develop a quality standard for the assessment, delivery and evaluation of spiritual care, ensuring a more consistent approach to the delivery of spiritual care. This type of inclusive approach to the development of spiritual assessment is an example of innovative practice and is central to contemporary UK government policy and guidance (Department of Health, 2008a, 2008b).

Practical aspects

The following quotation from Magee, Parsons and Askham can in my opinion be applied to the area of spiritual assessment and the delivery of spiritual care:

It is easier to make pronouncements about dignity than to ensure dignified care happens.

Magee, Parsons and Askham, 2008, p. 9

This quotation tells us that we can deliberate without any action being taken. It highlights the importance of action with regards to facilitating and ensuring that spiritual care is provided. Practical aspects cover all those finer details or features that are essential to the implementation of the 'ideal' spiritual assessment tool. The central features of a spiritual assessment tool are presented in Fig. 4.2. Catterall *et al.* write:

Assessment tools should be easy to use, flexible and take little time to assess the spiritual state of patients at different times and in different situations.

Catterall *et al.*, 1998, p. 4

Safety aspects

Safety must never be compromised. Therefore the construction and administration of any spiritual assessment tool must always safeguard and protect the patient/clients' safety, dignity, respect and confidentiality. It must be undertaken in an environment that upholds the integrity of the person. For example, it must not be undertaken in the middle of the ward with curtains drawn (although it is acknowledged that finding a private room free from interruption and distraction can be difficult) because we must remember that curtains are not barriers to sound and could result in a breach of confidentiality. Spiritual assessment is an enquiry into personal (and for some people, painful hidden) aspects of their lives which need to be handled sensitively and professionally and safely.

Figure 4.2   **Features of a spiritual assessment tool**

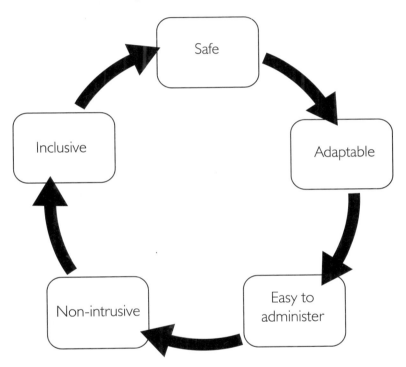

Attributes of spiritual assessment tools

Attributes of spiritual assessment

Adaptable

'Adaptable' means that a tool can be modified to suit different care contexts, and different client needs, while the term 'easily administered' refers to the ease with which a spiritual assessment can be undertaken. This should enable the practitioner and patient/client to feel comfortable and relaxed and it should be administered in a speedily uncomplicated manner. As stated earlier, a two-tiered approach may be used so that only patient/clients' religious needs are assessed upon admission. This may then be followed up with a more in-depth review. *We must also remember that some patients/clients may not want to enter into any dialogue about spiritual issues and this has to be respected.* The danger with developing spiritual assessment tools is that practitioners feel obliged to use them. The more assessments we develop the greater the risk of complicating care, and stifling skills of intuition and autonomy. Spiritual assessment tools must become an integral part of the admission and caring relationship.

Non-intrusive

Spiritual assessment tools must be constructed with sensitivity in mind and the introduction of any spiritual assessment must be undertaken with the full consent of the patient/client or with authorisation from their next of kin. This is fundamental when dealing with vulnerable adults and children. They must also be non-intrusive, meaning the questions should be non-threatening. The manner and timing of introducing any spiritual assessment tool is fundamental. Therefore the practitioner should be using all his or her professional skills to assess the patient/clients' physical and psychological status. For example a patient experiencing extreme pain or high levels of anxiety should not be subjected to lengthy questioning. McSherry and Ross (2002, p. 486) emphasise 'remembering it is an assessment, not an interrogation!'.

Inclusive

Inclusivity concerns the way the assessment has relevance to all groups receiving care within a specific healthcare context. It means close attention should be paid to the wording and language of the questions. The questions should be unambiguous and not alienate or discriminate between religious groups. This type of understanding will help to resolve some of the criticisms around spirituality being Judeo–Christian focused within healthcare contexts (Markham, 1998). The assessment should encourage active participation of all individuals in the entire assessment process. Particular attention should be given to the person undertaking the assessment, in that they should ensure that the process is conducted in a timely, non-intimidating and non-judgemental manner.

Who should undertake a spiritual assessment?

Who should undertake it?

There are several avenues of thought about who should undertake a spiritual assessment. In some areas this responsibility will be undertaken by a registered nurse since they are the professional group frequently involved in the admission process, especially within acute care settings. Yet an emerging model is the notion of spiritual care competencies ranging from level 1 through to level 4. Gordon and Mitchell indicate that practitioners operating at level 4 would be expected to demonstrate skills as described below:

> *Level 4 – Staff or volunteers whose primary responsibility is for the spiritual and religious care of patients, visitors and staff. Staff working at level 4 are expected to be able to manage and facilitate complex spiritual and religious needs in patients, families, carers, staff and volunteers, in particular the existential and practical needs arising from the impact on individuals and families from issues in illness, life, dying and death. In addition, they should have a clear understanding of their own personal beliefs.*

Gordon and Mitchell, 2004, p. 647

Irrespective of which model one adopts, the person undertaking the spiritual assessment should have sufficient training, have excellent awareness of their own spirituality and spiritual needs and be competent to deal with the issues that can transpire from such an interaction.

Ethical considerations

Ethical considerations

The introduction of any spiritual assessment must be undertaken with careful consideration. Cobb (1998, p. 117) alludes to the ethical issues when he writes: 'The hazards of assessing spiritual constructs are considerable'. Other writers talk about the ethics (Greenstreet, 2006) or ethical considerations when providing spiritual care (Farvis, 2005), while others address some of the ethical issues when outlining the barriers to providing spiritual care (Taylor, 2002). In my opinion it does not matter what language is used so long as the ethical issues are given sufficient thought and consideration. Ethical issues are important because they directly influence decision making in this area. Thought must be given to issues such as confidentiality, documentation and continuity of care. Issues of staffing and resources must also be adequately explored. Moreover, there are the issues of validity and reliability: does the tool measure what it is designed for and does it do this in a consistent manner (Cobb, 1998)? I would suggest that careful planning and development are critical factors in the design and planning processes.

Some of the hazards associated with spiritual assessment are explored in more depth within Chapter 8. Nevertheless I would like to illustrate the importance of 'ethics' with an anecdote from my own experience. I have attended several working groups charged with developing a spiritual assessment tool. Such groups are often comprised of enthusiastic, energetic and well-intentioned individuals who are assigned a specific brief in response to some form of policy or directive. While attending these groups I have raised questions about the purpose, education, training, support and potential impact of the spiritual assessment upon staff, patients/clients and the organisation. These ethical challenges are often met with some dismay; my questions are sometimes considered negative and unconstructive. Those charged with the development of such tools must grapple early on with some of these important ethical issues, to ensure they produce assessments that are suitable for purpose, context and patient/client group.

There is no good developing a spiritual assessment tool if practitioners (and I would add user groups), are not going to be consulted, or involved in the construction, implementation and ongoing evaluation. All staff must be sufficiently educated and introduced to the purpose and intended use of the spiritual assessment. Education will ensure spiritual assessment tools are used in an appropriate and competent manner. But more importantly, education will guarantee patients/clients are supported should any form of spiritual need be identified. The area of resource warrants mention. If spiritual assessments are introduced then there should be mechanisms to ensure that there are sufficiently qualified personnel with the correct skills to help support individuals. There should also be robust systems of governance to monitor impact and effectiveness, ensuring ongoing benefit for all.

Conclusion

This chapter introduced the different categories of spiritual assessment tools, drawing attention to some of the conceptual, organisational, practical and ethical challenges that must be considered by those developing and utilising them within healthcare contexts. I would like to conclude with a quotation from Cobb:

> ... as spirituality becomes rationalized and reduced to make it manageable, it begins to lose the subjective and specific human experience which makes it significant.
>
> Cobb, 1998, p. 117

Spiritual assessment must never detract from the humanistic and compassionate aspects of care. It must never be divisive or intrusive and it must always enhance care. There is also the danger that spiritual assessment and spiritual care will become fragmented and not integral to the delivery of care. It is recommended that patients and clients should identify their own sources of spiritual support, and the extent to which spiritual assessments are used must always be determined by the patient/client.

Spiritual assessment tools have the potential to enrich and promote the quality of patient care, but poorly constructed and utilised assessments could be counterproductive.

References

Anandarajah, G. and Hight, E. (2001). 'Spirituality and medical practice: Using the HOPE questions as a practical tool for spiritual assessment'. *American Family Physician*, 63(1), 81–88.

Burkhardt, M.A. and Nagai-Jacobson, M.G. (1985). 'Dealing with the spiritual concerns of clients in the community'. *Journal of Community Health Nursing*, 2, 191.

Carpenito, L.J. (1983). *Nursing Diagnosis: Application to Clinical Practice*. New York: JB Lippincott.

Carson, V.B. (1989). *Spiritual Dimensions of Nursing Practice*. Philadelphia: WB Saunders.

Catterall, R.A., Cox, M., Greet, B., Sankey, J. and Griffiths, G. (1998). 'The assessment and audit of spiritual care'. *International Journal of Palliative Nursing*, 4, 162–68.

Clarke, J. (2009). 'A critical view of how nursing has defined spirituality'. *Journal of Clinical Nursing*, **18**, 1666–73.

Cobb, M. (1998). 'Assessing spiritual needs: An examination of practice'. In: M. Cobb, V. Robshaw (eds) *The Spiritual Challenge of Healthcare*. Edinburgh: Churchill Livingstone.

Department of Health (2008a). *A High-Quality Workforce. NHS Next Stage Review*. London: Department of Health. Available from: http://www.dh.gov.uk/en/Healthcare/OurNHSourfuture/index.htm (last accessed April 2010).

Department of Health (2008b). *High-Quality Care for All. NHS Next Stage Review Final Report*. London: Department of Health: Available from: http://www.dh.gov.uk/en/Publicationsandstatistics/Publications/PublicationsPolicy AndGuidance/DH_085825 (last accessed April 2010).

Farvis, R.A. (2005). 'Ethical considerations in spiritual care'. *International Journal of Palliative Nursing*, **11**(4), 189.

Gilbert, P. (2008). *Guidelines on Spirituality for Staff in Acute Care Services*. London: National Institute for Mental Health in England.

Gordon, T. and Mitchell, D. (2004). 'A competency model for the assessment and delivery of spiritual care'. *Palliative Medicine*, **18**, 646–51.

Govier, I. (2000). 'Spiritual care in nursing: A systematic approach'. *Nursing Standard*, **14**, 32–36.

Greenstreet, W. (2006). *Integrating Spirituality in Health and Social Care*. Oxford: Radcliffe Publishing.

Highfield, M.F. (1993). 'PLAN: A spiritual care model for every nurse'. *Quality of Life*, **2**(3), 80–84.

Highfield, M.F. and Cason, C. (1983). 'Spiritual needs of patients: Are they recognised?' *Cancer Nursing*, **6**,187–92.

Hodge, D.R. (2001). 'Spiritual assessment: A review of major qualitative methods and a new framework for assessing spirituality'. *Social Work*, **46**(3), 203–14.

Hodge, D.R. (2005a). 'Spiritual lifemaps: A client-centered pictorial instrument for spiritual assessment, planning and intervention'. *Social Work*, **50**(1), 77–87.

Hodge, D.R. (2005b). 'Developing a spiritual assessment toolbox: A discussion of the strengths and limitations of five different assessment methods'. *Health and Social Work*, **30**(4), 314–23.

Hodge, D.R. (2006). 'A template for spiritual assessment: A review of the JCAHO requirements and guidelines for implementation'. *Social Work*, **51**(4), 317–26.

Human Rights Act (1998). Office of Public Sector Information. Available at: //http://www.opsi.gov.uk/acts/acts1998/ukpga_19980042_en_1 (last accessed April 2010).

Hunt, J., Cobb, M., Keeley, V.L. and Ahmedzia, S.H. (2003). 'The quality of spiritual care – developing a standard'. *International Journal of Palliative Nursing*, **9**(5), 208–15.

Koenig, H.G. (2002). *Spirituality in Patient Care Why, How, When and What*. Philadelphia: Templeton Foundation.

Ledger, S.D. (2005). The duty of nurses to meet patients' spiritual and/or religious needs. *British Journal of Nursing*, **14**(4), 220–25.

Magee, H., Parsons, S. and Askham, J. (2008). *Measuring Dignity in Care for Older People. A Research Report for Help the Aged*. London: Help the Aged.

Markham, I. (1998). 'Spirituality and the world faiths'. In: M. Cobb and V. Robshaw (eds) *The Spiritual Challenge of Healthcare*. Edinburgh: Churchill Livingstone, pp. 73–88.

Maugens, T.A. (1996). 'The SPIRITual history'. *Archives of Family Medicine*, **5**, 11–16.

McSherry, W. (2004). *The meaning of spirituality and spiritual care: An investigation of healthcare professionals', patients' and publics' perceptions*. PhD thesis. Leeds Metropolitan University.

McSherry, W. (2006). *Making Sense of Spirituality in Nursing and Healthcare Practice. An Interactive Approach*, 2nd edn. London: Jessica Kingsley.

McSherry, W. (2007). *The Meaning of Spirituality and Spiritual Care within Nursing and Healthcare Practice*. London: Quay Books.

McSherry, W. and Cash, K. (2004). 'The language of spirituality: An emerging taxonomy'. *International Journal of Nursing Studies*, **41**, 151–61.

McSherry, W. and Ross, L. (2002). 'Dilemmas of spiritual assessment: Considerations for nursing practice'. *Journal of Advanced Nursing*, **38**(5), 479–88.

Muncy, J.F. (1996). 'Muncy comprehensive spiritual assessment'. *The American Journal of Hospice and Palliative Care*, **13**, 44–45.

Narayanasamy, A. (1999). 'ASSET: A model for actioning spirituality and spiritual care education and training in nursing'. *Nurse Education Today*, **19**, 274–85.

Narayanasamy, A. (2001). *Spiritual Care: A Practical Guide for Nurses and Healthcare Practitioners*, 2nd edn. Wiltshire: Quay Books.

National Institute for Health and Clinical Excellence (2004). *Improving Supportive and Palliative Care for Adults with Cancer*. London: National Institute for Health and Clinical Excellence.

Nursing and Midwifery Council (2007). *Essential skills clusters (ESCs) for pre-registration nursing programmes. NMC Circular 07/2007*. London: NMC.

Paley, J. (2008). 'Spirituality and nursing: A reductionist approach'. *Nursing Philosophy*, **9**, 3–18.

Paley, J. (2009). 'Keep the NHS secular'. *Nursing Standard*, **23**(43), 26–27.

Pierce, B. (2004). 'The introduction and evaluation of a spiritual assessment tool in a palliative care unit'. *Scottish Journal of Healthcare Chaplaincy*, **7**(2), 39–43.

Puchalski, C. and Romer, A.L. (2000). 'Taking a spiritual history allows clinicians to understand patients more fully'. *Journal of Palliative Medicine*, **3**(1), 129–37.

Robinson, S., Kendrick, K. and Brown, A. (2003). *Spirituality and the Practice of Healthcare*. Hampshire: Palgrave Macmillan.

Roper, N., Logan, W. and Tierney, A. (1990). *The Elements of Nursing: A Model for Nursing Based on a Model of Living*, 3rd edn. Edinburgh: Churchill Livingstone.

Rumbold, B. (2002). *Spirituality and Palliative Care Social and Pastoral Perspective*. Australia: Oxford University Press.

Stoll, R. (1979). 'Guidelines for spiritual assessment'. *American Journal of Nursing*, 1, 1572–77.

Stoter, D. (1995). *Spiritual Aspects of Healthcare*. London: Mosby.

Swinton, J. (2001). *Spirituality and Mental Healthcare: Re-Discovering a 'Forgotten' Dimension*. London: Jessica Kingsley.

Tanyi, R.A. (2006). 'Spirituality and family nursing: spiritual assessment and interventions for families'. *Journal of Advanced Nursing*, **53**(3), 287–94.

Taylor, E.J. (2002). *Spiritual Care Nursing Theory, Research, and Practice*. New Jersey: Prentice Hall.

Timmins, F. and Kelly, J. (2008). 'Spiritual assessment in intensive and cardiac care nursing'. *Nursing in Critical Care*, **13**(3), 124–31.

van Leeuwen, R., Tiesinga, L.J., Middel, B., Post, D. and Jochemsen, H. (2009). 'The validity and reliability of an instrument to assess nursing competencies in spiritual care'. *Journal of Clinical Nursing*, **18**(20), 2857–69.

Chapter 5
The spiritual history: an essential element of patient-centred care

Christina Puchalski

Introduction

Spirituality is an essential element of healthcare because spirituality is, as Viktor Frankl wrote, the essence of our humanity (Frankl, 1963). It is that part of people that seeks healing, meaning and groundedness in the midst of suffering or illness (Foglio and Brody, 1988; Puchalski, 2002). Thus, broadly defined, spirituality is inclusive of non-believers as well as religious people. Atheist, agnostic, spiritual-but-not-religious and religious patients all have the desire for meaning and coherence. Illness or stress can disrupt the sense of meaning and purpose that all people strive for. Thus, spirituality can be a central issue for people that are ill or struggling with life's stresses.

There are several models used by healthcare professionals that support the inclusion of spirituality as a domain of the care of the patient. The biopsychosocial spiritual model (Sulmasy, 2002) describes the interconnectedness of all dimensions of care – physical, psychological, social (or psychosocial) and spiritual – in the care of patients. In this model, patients present with symptoms that may overlap in all four domains or may predominate in one more than the other. Thus pain or suffering may present as primarily physical or spiritual.

Patient-centred care is another model that supports the inclusion of spirituality in the care of patients. The Picker Institute notes that in patient-centred care, there are better healthcare outcomes if a patient's values and beliefs are respected. In the patient-centred care model there is recognition that a patient's understanding of illness can be impacted by many factors, including spiritual and religious beliefs and practices (Institute for Alternative Futures, 2004).

Spirituality and humanity

Spirituality and humanity

Spirituality, as an essential element of one's humanity, becomes central to any understanding the patient has about their inner life. Patient-centred care also describes the importance of how patients understand their illness in the context of their lives. Spiritual and religious beliefs have been shown to impact on understanding of illness as well as healthcare decisions (Phelps *et al.*, 2009; Puchalski, 2002). Finally, narrative medicine (Charon, 2001) illustrates the importance of eliciting and listening to patients' narratives – their life stories. Through the sharing of their stories, patients are able to realise what gives meaning to their lives. In the telling of their story, they celebrate their lives. Anecdotal evidence has shown that patients who share their personal perspective and stories about their views of illness and interpretation of life events can experience an integration of what is happening to them – a way to find healing in the midst of suffering and disease.

Intrinsic to patient narratives is the spiritual dimension of their lives. How does the patient find meaning and purpose? What are the significant experiences in their lives? What are the values that have guided their life and medical decisions? What resources help them in difficult times? How are they able to transcend suffering? What meaning does the illness hold for them? What legacy are they interested in leaving after their death?

Spirituality in the clinical setting

Spirituality in the clinical setting

Religious and spiritual themes arise often in the clinical setting. Some people might present with a sense of meaninglessness, or hopelessness; others might present with issues of forgiveness and/or resentment. Illness can trigger many spiritual issues and therefore the clinical setting may be the first place in which such issues arise. Religious issues can also cause distress in people's lives. Anger at 'their God' is common in the face of serious illness (the term 'their God' or 'her God' is used to denote a more multicultural perspective and an awareness of difference) and it can lead to conflict, guilt and despair. It is important in the clinical setting to allow people to talk about that anger in a safe environment where they do not feel they will be judged. In their religious communities they may be told that it is wrong to be angry at 'their God' or that it reflects a weakening in one's faith to be angry or feel abandoned, therefore the clinician's office may be a safe haven to explore these feelings in greater depth. Koenig and colleagues (Koenig *et al.*, 1998) found that negative religious coping was associated with poorer physical health, worse quality of life, and greater depression in medically ill hospitalised older adults, but positive religious coping was associated with better mental health. Understanding how spirituality and religion relate to patients' understanding of their illness and their ability to cope is an important aspect of providing comprehensive patient-centred care.

Patients' needs

Interestingly, there is also data that supports patients' requests for spiritual care from physicians and other healthcare professionals. Initial research suggests that between 41 and 94 per cent of patients want their physicians to address these issues. In one survey, even half of the non-religious patients thought that physicians should inquire politely about patients' spiritual needs (Ehman *et al.*, 1999). This is particularly true if patients are at the end of life, or are more religious to begin with. In numerous surveys, patients indicate their preference to have a more integrated approach to their care with their spiritual issues addressed by their healthcare professionals. In one study, 85 per cent of patients noted that their trust in their physician increases if that physician addresses their spiritual concerns (Ehman *et al.*, 1999). Ninety-five per cent of patients who report that spirituality is important want their doctor to be sensitive to their spiritual needs and to integrate it in their treatment. Fifty per cent of patients for whom spirituality is not important feel that physicians should address spiritual issues in the case of serious and chronic illness. In another study, McCord *et al.* (2004) reported that patients in a family practice setting again felt that it was important for physicians and healthcare providers to address their spiritual issues and beliefs. In this study, 95 per cent of patients wanted their spiritual beliefs considered in the case of serious illness, 86 per cent when admitted to a hospital, and 60 per cent during routine history taking.

Finally, in a survey of patients in hospital inpatient units, Astrow and colleagues found that the single most important predictor of satisfaction with care was whether the patient's spiritual needs were addressed in their care (Astrow *et al.*, 2007).

Communication about spiritual issues

The first step in communicating with patients about spiritual issues is to communicate a genuine interest and compassion for him or her. In a consensus conference sponsored by the Association of American Medical Colleges (AAMC) and the George Washington Institute for Spirituality and Health, medical educators, clinicians, medical ethicists and chaplains developed guidelines for spiritual care (Puchalski, 2006a).

Of particular importance was that clinicians should create environments in which patients feel they can trust their clinician and share whatever concerns they have, including their spiritual concerns. By creating an atmosphere of caring and compassion, as well as a willingness to be open to whatever is of concern to the patient, the interaction becomes focused in a patient-centred model of care. Thus the *first* step is to listen attentively with compassionate presence. The *second* step is to identify spiritual or religious themes in the conversation (National Comprehensive Cancer Network, 2008; Puchalski, 2002). These themes include:

- meaninglessness
- despair
- hopelessness
- religious distress
- conflict with religious/spiritual belief
- religious or spiritual ritual need
- reconciliation
- concerns with deity or transcendence
- concerns with the afterlife.

Some of the reasons for the resistance to addressing spirituality in the clinical setting include lack of time, lack of a clear definition of spirituality, or inappropriate clinician behaviour such as proselytising (Sloan *et al.*, 2000). Other reasons include the clinician's fear that inquiry into spiritual issues may trigger an existential crisis for the patient, which the clinician may not be trained to deal with or may not have the resources available to deal with it. However, as with any other part of the clinical history, issues may come up that the clinician does not have the expertise to deal with. Having experts on the interdisciplinary team, such as board-certified chaplains for spiritual care, helps provide the necessary care for following up on issues that the patient raises.

Stages in assessing spiritual issues

Communication with patients and families ranges from identification of spiritual issues to formal assessment of their spirituality (Lo *et al.*, 2002; Puchalski and Romer, 2000). There are four basic ways to approach communication about spiritual issues:

- recognition of spiritual themes, spiritual distress or suffering
- response to patient's statements about spiritual, religious or existential issues
- response to patient's cues
- formal spiritual history, screening or assessment.

The first three approaches can be applied by any member of the care team and are discussed below; the fourth stage is addressed independently in the next section (p. 87). During the clinical encounter, one should listen for expressions of spiritual themes and then follow up. For example, a patient may say 'I have no meaning' or 'What is the purpose of my life?' or may express a sense of hopelessness or despair in their conversations and behaviour. The clinician can ask the patient to explain more about these feelings and can then help identify appropriate treatment options. For example, with a patient who identifies a sense of meaningless in their life, the clinician could consider referral to a therapist or to meaning-oriented group therapy (Breitbart, 2003). For a patient who identifies a desire to seek a closer relationship to 'their God' or transcendence, the clinician can consider referral to a spiritual director. Or patients may express interest in yoga, meditation or some religious ritual. Remember that clinicians do not need to be experts in all spiritual or religious beliefs and practices; they can learn from their patients about what is important to them. Clinicians may be aware of resources in their community where they can refer patients for further information, such as a pastoral care department in the hospital, or a community yoga centre. If a patient wears religious or spiritual jewellery, or has religious or spiritual reading material at their bedside, clinicians can acknowledge them and ask questions about the significance of them.

A spiritual history, screening or assessment is a more formal part of the medical history in which the patient or the patient's family is asked about their spiritual and/or religious beliefs. In general, non-chaplain clinicians do a spiritual screening or a spiritual history; chaplains do a spiritual assessment. Spiritual screening or triage is a quick determination of whether a person is experiencing a serious spiritual crisis and therefore needs an immediate referral to a professional chaplain. Spiritual screening helps identify which patients may benefit from an in-depth spiritual assessment by a professional chaplain. Spiritual history-taking is the process of interviewing a patient about their spiritual beliefs and how those beliefs might impact upon their healthcare. The spiritual history questions are usually asked in the context of a comprehensive examination, by the clinician who is primarily responsible for providing direct care or referrals to specialists such as professional chaplains. Spiritual assessment refers to a more extensive assessment done by board-certified chaplains that is based on a narrative process. This assessment includes a spiritual care plan with expected outcomes, and plans for follow-up (Van de Creek and Lucas, 2001).

In hospitals, nursing homes, or hospices, the nurse or social worker upon triage or admission does the spiritual screening. The purpose is to access for spiritual emergencies that may require a chaplain immediately. Once the initial admission process is complete, a spiritual history is taken as part of the complete history carried out by physicians or nurses, or social workers who see the patient after the initial triage. In outpatient settings, the process may differ. If the patient comes to the physician's office and is in distress, a spiritual screening might be done as part of the initial conversation with the physician, nurse practitioner, or physician-assistant. Screening for spiritual distress might also occur in the context of the spiritual history.

Regardless of the setting, all patients should have their spiritual issues addressed in the context of their care. Chaplains are the spiritual care specialists while other clinicians function as generalists in spiritual care. Thus all clinicians recognise and address spiritual issues with patients; they also should refer to chaplains for more intense assessment and treatment as needed.

Spiritual history tools

**Spiritual
history tools**

For non-chaplains, the spiritual history can be integrated into the intake history, usually as part of the social history. A spiritual history is as important as any other part of the clinical history. When doing a clinical history, clinicians target specific areas. Simply listening to themes alone will not elicit all the information needed to provide good medical care. This is why specific questions need to be asked, in order to target areas of information regarding depression, social support, sexuality, domestic violence, smoking and alcohol or drug use. A spiritual history is simply a set of targeted questions aimed at inviting patients to share their spiritual and/or religious beliefs if desired and to guide them to share their thoughts about their meaning in their life particularly as it relates to what is happening to them in the clinical setting (for example, a new diagnosis or loss or other life stress).

Preliminary questions can be used to invite patients to share their thoughts about their spirituality. Several tools have been developed for this purpose. These include FICA (Puchalski and Romer, 2000; Puchalski, 2006b), SPIRIT (Maugans, 1996) and HOPE (Anandarajah and Hight, 2001) as summarised in Box 5.1 (p. 88). These tools include spiritual or religious identification, the importance of the belief and the way the beliefs affect healthcare decision-making, and what community affiliation the patient has. The FICA tool is the only one that has been validated (Borneman *et al.*, in press). It appears here in a slightly modified form, but when using it to interview patients the language in the original version should be used. This can be accessed on the GWish web site (www.gwish.org) where you can also view a video on how to use it.

The questions outlined in these tools are meant to serve as a guide for the discussion about spiritual issues. This framework, and the questions accompanying it, can be customised to be consistent with the patient's or client's orientation and needs. For example, if the patient is coming for a routine visit, one might address spirituality in the context of stress management or health. If the patient has just been told of a serious diagnosis, then the questions might be phrased differently. For example: 'Do you have spiritual beliefs that have helped you in difficult times before?' or 'It must be hard to hear difficult news like this – do you have any spiritual beliefs that might help you right now?'.

Box 5.1

Taking a spiritual history according to (a) FICA (based on Puchalski and Romer, 2000; Puchalski, 2006b; Puchalski *et al.*, 2009; to which the reader is referred), **(b) SPIRIT** (based on Maugens, 1997) **and (c) HOPE** (based on Anandarajah and Hight, 2001).

(a) FICA

F FAITH and belief
Does the patient consider him- or herself to be spiritual or religious?[1] Or:
Does the patient have spiritual beliefs that help him or her cope with stress?[1]
If the patient answers 'No', ask: 'What gives your life meaning?''
(Ask about 'meaning' even if the patient answers 'Yes').

I IMPORTANCE [2]
What importance does this faith or belief have in the patient's life?
Have these beliefs influenced how the patient takes care of him- or herself during the illness?
What role do these beliefs play in the patient's health?
Do these beliefs affect any of the patient's healthcare decisions?

C COMMUNITY
Is the patient part of a spiritual or religious community? Is this of support to the patient? How?[3]
Is there a group of people the patient really loves or who are important to the patient?

A ADDRESS in care or action[4]
How would the patient like the healthcare provider to address these issues in his or her healthcare? Or:
What action or steps does the patient need to take in his or her spiritual journey?

(b) SPIRIT

S SPIRITUAL belief system
Does the patient have a formal religious affiliation and, if so, can he or she describe it?
Does the patient have a spiritual life that is important to him or her?
What gives the patient the clearest sense of meaning in his or her life?

P PERSONAL spirituality
Which beliefs and practices of your religion does the patient personally accept and which beliefs and practices are not accepted or followed?
In what ways is the patient's spirituality/religion meaningful to him or her?
How is the patient's spirituality/religion important in his or her daily life?

I INTEGRATION with a spiritual community
Does the patient belong to any religious or spiritual groups or communities?
How does the patient participate in this group or community and, if so, in what role?
What importance does this group have for the patient and in what ways is this a source of support?
What type of support and help does or could this group provide for the patient in dealing with health issues?

R **RITUALISED** practices and restrictions

What specific practices does the patient carry out as part of his or her religious and spiritual life (e.g. prayer, meditation or attending a service)?

What lifestyle activities or practices does the patient's religion encourage, discourage or forbid?

What meaning do these practices and restrictions have for the patient, and to what extent has he or she followed these guidelines?

I **IMPLICATIONS** for medical care

Are there specific elements of medical care that the patient's religion discourages or forbids, and to what extent has he or she followed these guidelines?

What aspects of this religion/spirituality would the patient like to keep in mind as he or she is cared for?

What knowledge or understanding would strengthen the patient's relationship with the healthcare provider?

Are there barriers to the patient's relationship with those caring for his or her health right now that are based upon religious or spiritual issues?

Would the patient like to discuss any religious or spiritual implications of healthcare?

T **TERMINAL** events planning

Are there particular aspects of medical care the patient wishes to avoid or to have withheld because of his or her religion/spirituality?

Are there any religious/spiritual practices or rituals the patient would like to have available in the hospital or at home?

Are there religious/spiritual practices the patient wishes to plan for at the time of his or her death or after death?

From what sources does the patient draw strength in order to cope with this illness?

(c) HOPE

H HOPE

What are the patient's sources of hope, strength, comfort, meaning, peace, love and connection?

O ORGANISED religion

What role does organised religion have for the patient?

P PERSONAL

What is the patient's personal spirituality and what practices does this involve?

E EFFECTS

What are the effects of the patient's spirituality/beliefs on their medical care and end-of-life decisions?

1 Contextualise to the situation (e.g. with what he or she is going through right now, with dying and dealing with pain).

2 These questions can help lead to others about advance directives and proxies who can represent the patient's beliefs and values. Also ask about spiritual practices and rituals that might be important.

3 Communities such as churches, temples, mosques, family or a group of like-minded friends can provide strong support systems.

4 Often it is not necessary to ask these questions – instead think about which spiritual issues need to be addressed in the treatment plan, for example referral to a chaplain, a pastoral counsellor or a spiritual director, keeping a journal or music or art therapy. Sometimes the plan may be simply to listen and support the patient in his or her journey.

As mentioned above, the spiritual history is normally done during the social history section of the initial assessment as one is asking the patient about their living situation and significant relationships. The clinician can transition into finding out how the person cares for him or herself. Just as questions about exercise and how one deals with stress and difficult situations are an important part of self-care, questions about the importance of spiritual beliefs and practices should be included. The spiritual history might also be taken in specific clinical situations where spiritual issues arise, for example in breaking bad news, or in end-of-life situations. The spiritual history should also be taken at follow-up visits as appropriate. Box 5.2 presents the spiritual history within the clinical context.

Box 5.2

Things to include in the social history section of an initial interview

- Important relationships, marital status, significant other, etc.
- Sexual history
- Occupational history
- Avocation
- Risk assessment (smoking, alcohol or drug usage, not wearing a seat belt, domestic violence)
- Wellness/prevention (exercise, nutrition, emotional well-being, spiritual history)

A spiritual history involves more than simply asking questions. First, it is important to create an environment of trust so that the patient knows that what they may share will be respected. Second, it is critical to be open to listening to the patient's story – not just facts. Hence, what someone shares about meaning and purpose or despair needs to be attended to with compassionate presence and full attention. Anecdotally, medical students have often observed that 'something in the room changes' when they ask patients their spiritual history. Being present can open up the possibility of what some consider to be a healing encounter. The very act of providing the patient space to share about his or her beliefs and feelings gives them the opportunity to find resources of strength within themselves and possibly ways of better coping with suffering and finding inner healing.

Given the intimacy of the clinical encounter, where the patient shares issues of meaning, suffering, and deep feelings, it is important that the clinician honours the dignity of the patient at all times. In any aspect of the clinical encounter it is critical to recognise that there is a marked power imbalance between the clinician and the patient. Clinicians have an obligation to respect patients and to do only that which is in the best interest of the patient. Thus, it would be absolutely unethical to proselytise patients with the clinician's belief system or to ridicule patients about their beliefs or about a lack of scientific validity in belief systems (if that is what the clinician believes).

Respect, patient-centredness, and inclusivity are three key ethical principles that can guide and underpin medical practice (Canda and Furman, 1999; Nelson-Becker *et al.*, 2006). Respect means to value the patient's view, even if it seems unorthodox or different from the clinician's views. It means to respect the patient's desire for privacy in all matters, including the spiritual, and to give the patient assurance that anything the patient shares will be held in confidence and will not be ridiculed or ignored.

Integrating spirituality into the care plan

Spirituality and the care plan

Once the clinician identifies a spiritual issue, the clinician then decides how to integrate that into the treatment or care plan. There a several models for how to do this, which resulted from a national consensus initiative to develop spiritual care guidelines (Puchalski *et al.*, 2009). Ideally, an interdisciplinary team of healthcare professionals, which includes a board-certified chaplain as the spiritual care expert, develops the treatment or care plan. If there is no interdisciplinary team, for example in an outpatient setting, the clinician needs to work with spiritual care professionals such as an outpatient chaplain, pastoral counsellor or spiritual director or community clergy, religious leaders or culturally-based healers.

The information gathered from the spiritual history needs to be documented in the patient's medical chart or electronic database. One way to do this is to follow the biopsychosocial–spiritual model and document the assessment and plan in that holistic framework (Puchalski, 2002). An example of this is shown in the case described in Case Example 5.1.

Case example 5.1

An 80-year-old man is dying of end-stage colon cancer with well-controlled pain but some anxiety, unresolved family issues, and fear about dying. Using the biopsychosocial–spiritual model of Puchalski (2007) he can be assessed according to the following four dimensions and an appropriate treatment plan can be devised.

PHYSICAL: Assessment shows that his pain is well controlled. He is still having episodes of nausea and vomiting, probably secondary to partial small bowel obstruction. Continue with his current medication regimen and evaluate the treatment options to relieve any nausea associated with bowel obstruction.

EMOTIONAL: Assessment shows he has anxiety about dyspnoea, which may be associated with dying. The anxiety is affecting his sleep at night. Refer him to a counsellor for anxiety management and to explore any issues about fear of dying. Consider a palliative care consultation for treatment of dyspnoea and anxiety.

SOCIAL: Assessment shows he has unresolved issues with certain family members, as well as questions about funeral planning and costs. Refer him to a social worker for possible family intervention as well as assistance with end-of-life planning.

SPIRITUAL: Assessment allows him to express his fears about dying and the fact that he is seeking forgiveness from his son for being a 'distant dad'. Consider referring him to a chaplain for spiritual counselling. Consider forgiveness intervention regarding his son. Encourage discussion with him about his fear of death. Continue to provide your presence and support.

In addition, when patients leave a hospital or other inpatient setting, the discharge plan should also include the holistic model. Thus, if there are spiritual issues, these should be included in the discharge plan with the appropriate follow-up as indicated in the case described in Case Example 5.2.

Case example 5.2

A 65-year-old woman is admitted for repair of a hip fracture. The surgery went well, without complications, and now she being discharged to a rehabilitation facility. It has been noted that she is experiencing anxiety, and has been separated from her religious community. She has strong spiritual beliefs, a good level of hope and strong family support. Her spiritual goal includes deepening her relationship with 'her God'. She has expressed an interest in learning meditation. Using the biopsychosocial–spiritual discharge plan (Puchalski et al., 2009) her problems can be addressed according to the following four dimensions, and appropriate treatment can be planned.

PHYSICAL: Her status post hip fracture requires physical and occupational therapy. Ensure she receives adequate pain management.

EMOTIONAL: She is anxious about not being able to work, and she has panic attacks at night. Evaluate the options to treat her anxiety and sleeplessness. These might include counselling with a social worker.

SOCIAL: She is isolated in a new facility. Encourage her family to visit her and contact rehabilitation services for information regarding activities, volunteers and other available support.

SPIRITUAL: She has become isolated from her church community, yet she desires to deepen her relationship with 'her God'. Referral to a chaplain will help, and consider referral to spiritual director once she is discharged from rehab. Provide a list of meditation centres and teachers in her community or refer her to social work for basic instruction.

Conclusion

Patient-centred care is based on the principle that the focus of care is on the patient not just on their disease. Thus, any clinical history should have questions directed at all aspects of the patient's life, including the spiritual. The main purpose of the spiritual history is to listen to the patient's spiritual narrative and to give him or her the opportunity to share thoughts about their hopes, despairs, meaning and what is of importance to them. It allows the clinician to signal to the patient that the clinician respects them and is willing to listen to whatever is of value or concern to him or her. By asking 'Are you spiritual?' or 'What gives your life meaning?' the clinician is also saying: 'I am interested in you as a person and interested in the way you are coping with your illness and finding meaning in your life'. It says to the patient that the care he or she will receive is not just about the physical, but also about psychosocial and spiritual aspects. It acknowledges the importance of whole-person care that focuses on the illness as part of the patient's life-story and not just his or her disease.

References

Anandarajah, G. and Hight, E. (2001). 'Spirituality and medical practice: Using the HOPE questions as a practical tool for spiritual assessment'. *American Family Physician*, **63**(1), 81–89.

Astrow, A.B., Wexler, A., Texeira, K., Kai He, M., and Sulmasy, D.P. (2007). 'Is failure to meet spiritual needs associated with cancer patients' perceptions of quality of care and their satisfaction with care?' *Journal of Clinical Oncology*, **25**(36), 5753–57.

Borneman, T., Ferrell, B. and Puchalski, C. (in press). 'Evaluation of the FICA tool for spiritual assessment'. *Journal of Pain and Symptom Management*.

Breitbart, W. (2003). 'Reframing hope: Meaning-centred care for patients near the end of life. Interview by Karen S. Heller'. *Journal of Palliative Medicine*, **6**(6), 979–88.

Canda, E.R., and Furman, L.D. (1999). *Spiritual Diversity in Social Work Practice: The Heart of Helping*. New York: Free Press.

Charon, R. (2001). 'Narrative medicine: A model for empathy, reflection, profession, and trust'. *Journal of the American Medical Association*, **286**(15), 1897–1902.

Ehman, J.W., Ott, B.B., Short, T.H., Ciampa, R.C. and Hansen-Flaschen, J. (1999). 'Do patients want physicians to inquire about their spiritual or religious beliefs if they become gravely ill?' *Archives of Internal Medicine*, **159**(15), 1803–06.

Foglio, J.P. and Brody, H. (1988). 'Religion, faith, and family medicine'. *Journal of Family Practice*, **27**(5), 473–74.

Frankl, V.E. (1963). *Man's Search for Meaning*. New York, NY: Washington Square Press, Simon and Schuster.

Institute for Alternative Futures (2004). *Patient-Centred Care, 2015: Scenarios, Vision, Goals and Next Steps*. Alexandria, VA: The Picker Institute.

Koenig, H.G., Pargament, K.I. and Nielson, J. (1998). 'Religious coping and health status in medically ill hospitalised older adults'. *The Journal of Nervous and Mental Disease*, **186**(9), 513–21.

Lo, B., Ruston, D., Kates, L.W., *et al.* (2002). 'Discussing religious and spiritual issues at the end of life: A practical guide for physicians'. *Journal of the American Medical Association*, **287**(6), 749–54.

Maugans, T.A. (1996). 'The SPIRITual history'. *Archives of Family Medicine*, **5**(1), 11–16.

McCord, G., Gilchrist, V.J., Grossman, S.D., *et al.* (2004). 'Discussing spirituality with patients: A rational and ethical approach'. *Annals of Family Medicine*, **2**(4), 356–61.

National Comprehensive Cancer Network (2008). *NCCN Clinical Practice Guidelines in Oncology: Distress Management*. Available at: http://www.nccn.org/professionals/physician_gls/PDF/distress.pdf.

Nelson-Becker, H., Nakashima, M. and Canda, E.R. (2006). 'Spirituality in professional helping interventions with older adults'. In: B. Berkman and S. Ambruoso (eds) *Oxford Handbook of Social Work in Health and Aging*. New York: Oxford University Press, pp. 797–807.

Phelps, A.C., Maciejewski,, P.K., Nilsson, M., *et al.* (2009). 'Religious coping and use of intensive life-prolonging care near death in patients with advanced cancer'. *Journal of the American Medical Association*, **301**(11), 1140–47.

Puchalski, C. (2002). 'Spirituality'. In: A. Berger, R. Portenoy and D. Weissman (eds) *Principles and Practice of Palliative Care and Supportive Oncology*, 2nd edn. Philadelphia: Lippincott Williams and Wilkins, pp. 799–812.

Puchalski, C. (2006a). 'Spirituality and medicine: Curricula in medical education'. *Journal of Cancer Education*, **21**(1), 14–18.

Puchalski, C. (2006b). 'Spiritual assessment in clinical practice'. *Psychiatric Annals*, **36**(3), 150.

Puchalski, C. (2007). 'Spirituality and the care of patients at the end-of-life: An essential component of care'. *Omega Journal of Death and Dying*, **56**(1), 33–46.

Puchalski, C. and Romer, A.L. (2000). 'Taking a spiritual history allows clinicians to understand patients more fully'. *Journal of Palliative Medicine*, **3**(1), 129–37.

Puchalski, C., Ferrell, B., Virani, R., Otis-Green, S., Baird, P. and Bull, J. (2009). 'Improving the quality of spiritual care as a dimension of palliative care: Consensus conference report'. *Journal of Palliative Medicine*, **12**(10), 885–904.

Sloan, R.P., Bagiella, E., Van de Creek, L., *et al.* (2000). 'Should physicians prescribe religious activity?' *New England Journal of Medicine*, **342**(25), 1913–16.

Sulmasy, D.P. (2002). 'A biopsychosocial–spiritual model for the care of patients at the end of life'. *Gerontologist*, **42**(3), 24–33'.

Van de Creek, L. and Lucas, A.M. (2001). *The Discipline for Pastoral Care Giving: Foundations for Outcome Oriented Chaplaincy*. New York: Haworth Pastoral Press.

Chapter 6
Indicator-based and value clarification tools

Donia Baldacchino

Introduction

In earlier chapters the concepts of spirituality and spiritual need were explored. In Chapter 5 some examples of spiritual assessment tools for use in clinical practice were described. Reference to the extensive body of research into spirituality has been mentioned throughout the book so far, emphasising this growing field of academic and scholarly enquiry. Now this chapter will focus on the sorts of tools and instruments that may be useful in researching spirituality, by seeking to answer the following key questions:

- What aspect or aspects of spirituality or spiritual care do these scales and instruments measure?
- Why is there a need to measure these aspects of spirituality?
- What do they contribute to understanding?
- How do these scales and measures assist researchers and educators?

Consequently, this chapter has a more academic style than previous ones and it will be of particular interest to those conducting research in this field as well as educators seeking to develop awareness of the diverse attitudes that might be held about spirituality.

Enquiry into spirituality

Earlier discussions have revealed that the concepts of spirituality, spiritual well-being and spiritual care are multidimensional and very complex. This presents a major challenge to those who are enquiring into these concepts, whether using quantitative or qualitative research methods (Box 6.1).

Irrespective of which research method is used, neither can reveal the true nature of these concepts. Therefore, the use of scales or tools will at best only provide indicators that reflect the constituents of the concept rather than the phenomenon itself (Polit and Beck, 2006). Thus, the 'scores' obtained are subjective indicators of the concept addressed, particularly if the tools have only a small number of items (Boero *et al.*, 2005). Additionally, research tools rely on inferences made from statistical information derived from psychometric testing which contribute towards the reliability and validity of the instrument (Polit and Hungler, 1999).

Box 6.1

Distinguishing between quantitative and qualitative research

Quantitative

    Numerical data and statistical tests

    Measurement tools and scales

Qualitative

    People's views, experiences and understandings

    Interview transcripts, observations, diaries

Seven facets of spirituality

Seven facets of spirituality

This chapter will focus upon the quantitative measures developed to measure seven facets of spirituality (the number of measures presented for each facet are given in brackets). These are:

1. Spirituality as a concept in its own right (n = 6).

2. Spiritual well-being (n = 5).

3. Spiritual needs (n = 2).

4. Meaning and purpose in life (n = 4).

5. Spiritual coping (n = 2).

6. Spirituality as part of quality of life (n = 1).

7. Spiritual care (n = 4).

Identification of the scales

Identification of the scales

The above facets and their corresponding research instruments were derived from an extensive review of literature from 1975 to 2009 (the end of the literature search was 30 July 2009) on the following databases: EBSCO, PubMed, CINAHL (Cumulative Index to Nursing and Allied Health Literature) and BioMed Central. The keywords used included a combination of the following: assessment, measure, tool, instrument, scale, spirituality, spiritual coping, spiritual well-being, spiritual health, spiritual needs and spiritual care.

The tools presented in this chapter are not an exhaustive list because some literature could not be obtained or it was available but it did not contain the necessary psychometric values, for example, the Index of Core Spiritual Experiences (INSPIRIT; Kass *et al.*, 1991); the Spirituality Assessment Scale (SAS; Howden, 1992); the Spiritual Needs Related to Illness Tool (SPIRIT; Taylor, 2006); and the Meaning in Life Scale (MiLS; Jim *et al.*, 2006). Twenty-four tools are presented, which satisfied the following criteria:

- addressing reliability and validity testing of the tool
- assessing spirituality as a whole or characteristics of spirituality such as self-transcendence, finding meaning and purpose in life
- measuring spirituality which may incorporate religiosity
- investigating spiritual well-being and spiritual care.

Tools that viewed spirituality as being synonymous with religion were excluded.

These tools offer insights into the diverse perceptions and understandings that people may hold regarding spirituality within different contexts. The seven facets of spirituality outlined above and their selected measures will be presented using the following format.

Format and presentation of the scales and measures

- Title: Name given to measuring instrument or scale.
- Example: An example of where and how the scale has been used in a research investigation or in some instances how the scale was developed.
- Country of origin: Where the scale was developed.

- Developmental participants: Subjects included in development of the scale.

- Description of scale: The number of questions or items included in the scale, and the number of response options.

- Factors: The elements that are measured by a particular scale. The number of factors identified that demonstrate the construct validity of the tool.

- Overall consistency: The value of Cronbach alpha coefficient which denotes the extent of internal consistency of the tool. The nearer the value to 1.00 the higher the degree of homogeneity of the scale (Polit and Beck, 2006).

Seven facets of spirituality explored

Facet 1: Spirituality as a concept in its own right

Seven facets explored

Within this section, six measures were identified addressing diverse aspects of spirituality, suggesting that spirituality is personal, is associated with individual belief, the notion of transcendence, religiosity, and how people exert control over their lives. Collectively the measures imply that spirituality integrates the biopsychosocial dimensions and may or may not include the religious dimension, depending upon the individual's belief system. For the believer, religiosity may play an important role in coping with illness (Baldacchino, 2003; Koenig *et al.*, 2001). Diversity and individualism may still persist, even when individuals hold the same fixed religion (McSherry *et al.*, 2004; Swinton and Narayanasamy, 2002). The ultimate outcome of spirituality is to find personal meaning and purpose in life (Bauer-Wu and Farran, 2005; Frankl, 1962).

1. **Spirituality Self-rating Scale (SSRS)** (Galanter *et al.*, 2007)

- *Country of origin*: USA

- *Description of scale*: Six items on a five-point Likert-form scale (Strongly agree–Strongly disagree)

- *Developmental participants*: Healthy non-substance abusers (n = 352) and substance abusers (n = 473)

- *Factors*: One (spiritual orientation to life)

- *Overall internal consistency*: Cronbach alpha 0.82–0.91

Example: Galanter *et al.* (2007) investigated differences in spiritual orientation to life between healthy non-substance abusers, namely medical students (n = 119), university students (n = 180), medical addiction faculty (n = 34); Chaplaincy trainees (n = 19), and various groups of substance abusers on rehabilitation programmes (dually diagnosed psychiatric inpatients (n = 101), therapeutic community residents (n = 210), patients on methadone maintenance (n = 110) and methadone anonymous members (n = 52)). The substance abusers were significantly more spiritual than the students. This implies that spirituality is an important motivator for substance-dependent persons on rehabilitation programmes.

2. Spiritual Involvement and Beliefs Scale–Revised (SIBS–R)
(Hatch *et al.*, 1998)

- *Country of origin*: USA
- *Description of scale*: Twenty-six items on a seven-point Likert-form scale (Strongly agree–Strongly disagree)
- *Developmental participants*: Adults affiliated with Christianity, Judaism, Islam, Hinduism (n = 393)
- *Factors*: Two (religious practices and beliefs; spiritual practices and beliefs)
- *Overall internal consistency*: Cronbach alpha 0.83

Example: Arevalo *et al.* (2008) examined the role of spirituality, sense of coherence, and coping responses in relation to stress and trauma symptoms in 393 women undertaking a substance abuse treatment programme. A negative significant relationship was found between perceived stress and spirituality, sense of coherence, and coping. It implies that substance abuse treatment programmes appear to increase spirituality, which may decrease levels of stress and post-traumatic stress symptoms. Thus underlining the importance of including the spiritual dimension in rehabilitation programmes in order to enhance adjustment and compliance.

3. Spiritual Transcendence Index (STI) (Seidlitz *et al.*, 2002)

- *Country of origin*: USA
- *Description of scale*: Eight items on a six-point Likert-form scale (Extremely disagree–Extremely agree)
- *Developmental participants*: College students (n = 113)
- *Factors*: Two (spirituality; religiosity)
- *Overall internal consistency*: Cronbach alpha 0.86

Example: Kim and Seidlitz (2002) investigated relationship between spirituality and emotional and physical adjustment to daily stress of 113 college students undertaking an introductory psychology course in Seoul, Korea. Spirituality was found to buffer the adverse effects of stress and contributed to their adjustment to the new programme. Thus, spirituality needs to be incorporated in preventive programmes in order to enhance students' coping.

4. Brief Multidimensional Measure of Religiousness/Spirituality (BMMRS) (Fetzer Group/National Institute on Aging working group (1999))

- *Country of origin*: USA
- *Description of scale*: Four-point Likert-form scale (not cited)
- *Developmental participants*: Patients with musculoskeletal pain (n = 122)
- *Factors*: Eleven domains (daily spiritual experiences; values/beliefs; forgiveness; private religious practices; religious and spiritual coping; religious support; religious/spiritual history; commitment; organisational religiousness; religious preference; overall self-ranking)
- *Overall internal consistency*: Cronbach alpha 0.54–0.91

Example: Rippentrop *et al.* (2005) investigated the relationship between religiousness/spirituality and physical and mental health on 122 patients with chronic musculoskeletal pain. A negative significant relationship was found between religiousness and poor physical health. This indicates that patients experiencing low physical health were more likely to use religious coping strategies such as prayer and meditation. In contrast, patients with chronic pain felt more abandoned by God. Therefore, religion/spirituality may have a positive or negative impact on patients. Thus, assessment of patients' multidimensional spirituality is needed in order to address their holistic needs.

5. Expression of Spirituality Inventory (ESI) (MacDonald, 2000)

- *Country of origin*: USA
- *Description of scale*: Ninety-eight items on a five-point Likert-form scale (1–5)
- *Developmental participants*: University undergraduate students (n = 296)
- *Factors*: Five (cognitive orientation towards spirituality;

experiential/phenomenological dimension; existential well-being; beliefs; religiousness)

● *Overall internal consistency*: Cronbach alpha 0.85–0.97

Example: MacDonald investigated the relationship between spirituality and boredom proneness in 296 university undergraduate students. Existential well-being was identified as the strongest predictor of boredom proneness for both men and women. This is consistent with the finding of a negative significant correlation between existential well-being and boredom proneness for both genders. Thus, individuals who manage to find meaning and purpose in life are less liable to experience boredom.

6. Spiritual Health Locus of Control Scale (Holt *et al*, 2007)

● *Country of origin*: USA

● *Description of scale*: Number of items not given. Five-point Likert-form scale (Strongly agree–Strongly disagree)

● *Developmental participants*: Women (n = 112)

● *Factors*: Two (internal health locus of control; external health locus of control)

● *Overall internal consistency*: Cronbach alpha 0.52

Example: Holt *et al*. (2007) investigated the relationships between spirituality and locus of control on 112 African–American women participating in the educational intervention project for breast cancer. A positive correlation was found between active spirituality and faith in God's grace and internal locus of control. In contrast, passive spirituality was positively related with external locus of control. These findings are consistent with Rotter's social learning theory (Rotter, 1966) whereby individuals with internal locus of control believe that they have control over their own outcomes. In contrast, those with an external locus of control believe that their outcomes are controlled by outside forces such as luck, chance, fate or powerful others.

Facet 2: Spiritual well-being

Within this section five spiritual well-being scales are presented. Spiritual well-being is defined by Hungelmann *et al*. as:

> ... *a sense of harmonious interconnectedness between self, others/nature, and Ultimate Other which exists throughout and*

beyond time and space. It is achieved through a dynamic and integrative growth process which leads to a realisation of the ultimate purpose and meaning of life.
Hungelmann *et al.*, 1985, p. 152

Hungelmann *et al.* (1985) broadened the definition to include the views of atheists. While atheists did not believe in a Supreme Being, the believers' connection consisted of a relationship with God by their love and trust in Him, achieved through prayer and worship. In addition, inner harmony could be achieved by satisfaction with self and acceptance of the limitations in life situations together with a positive attitude and self-determination to maintain inner peace even during crises. The outcome of spiritual well-being is finding meaning and purpose in life, self-transcendence and guiding values for problem-solving, even in times of illness. This is consistent with research whereby pivotal events such as an illness may encourage and enable individuals to increase their spiritual well-being (Baldacchino, 2003; Koenig *et al.*, 2001).

1. Index of Spiritual Well-being (Moberg, 1979)

- *Country of origin*: USA
- *Description of scale*: Number of items not given. Four-point Likert-form scale (Yes–Don't know)
- *Developmental participants*: Sociology research students (n = 121)
- *Factors*: Three (beliefs about spiritual well-being; characteristics of spiritual well-being; influences on spiritual well-being)
- *Overall internal consistency*: Cronbach alpha not given

Example: Moberg (1979) explored spiritual well-being of 121 students undertaking sociological research module in USA. The findings showed the characteristics of spiritual well-being, namely finding meaning in life, having harmony with self, happiness, and being good to others. Those students who rated themselves as having spiritual well-being ranked religious items more highly than others, such as peace with God and faith in Christ. The students reported that their spiritual well-being was influenced by their friends, family, personal crises such as illness, the death of a relative or friend, and receiving Holy Communion. The students identified a distinction between organised religion and spiritual practices, both of which may contribute towards spiritual well-being. This study provided insight on the spiritual dimension in life and generated further quantitative and qualitative research.

2. Spiritual Well-being Scale (Paloutzian and Ellison, 1991)

- *Country of origin*: USA
- *Description of scale*: Twenty items on a six-point Likert-form scale (Strongly agree–Strongly disagree)
- *Developmental participants*: USA students from religious-oriented colleges (n = 206)
- *Factors*: Two (religious well-being; existential well-being)
- *Overall internal consistency*: Cronbach alpha 0.76–0.81

Example: Witt Sherman *et al.* (2005) investigated relationships between spiritual well-being and quality of life (QOL) on 206 patients with advanced cancer and AIDS aged 18 years and over and their family caregivers. Findings showed similarities in spiritual well-being scores among AIDS and cancer patients, indicating that the spiritual needs of patients at the end of life may be similar, irrespective of the type of illness. This is supported by McClain-Jacobson *et al.* (2004) who found that spirituality has a powerful psychological effect on patients with advanced cancer.

3. Jarel Spiritual Well-being Scale (Hungelmann *et al.*, 1985)

- *Country of origin*: USA
- *Description of scale*: Twenty-one items on a six-point Likert-form scale (Strongly agree–Strongly disagree)
- *Developmental participants*: Older adults of mean age 73 years (n = 294)
- *Factors*: Three (faith/belief; life/self-responsibility; life satisfaction/self-actualisation)
- *Overall internal consistency*: Cronbach alpha 0.85

Example: Hungelmann *et al.* (1989) assessed spiritual well-being in 294 older persons aged 65–97 years old, recruited from across the health-illness continuum from a variety of settings. The majority were women (238). The findings denoted that harmony in life consisted of satisfaction in relationships of the past and present, interconnection oriented towards mutual relationships and self-growth over time, and hope for the future. Spiritual well-being could be an internal resource of coping in life situations. This was supported by Baldacchino (2002) who investigated spiritual well-being, anxiety and depression on a sample of 70 patients from Malta (46 men and 24 women, aged 40–89) during the first three months after acute myocardial infarction. The scores of spiritual well-being were maintained at a high level across time. Thus, it appears that spiritual well-being is an internal resource of coping that may contribute towards the decline of anxiety and depression across time.

4. Spiritual Health And Life Orientation Measure (Shalom) (Fisher, 1999)

- *Country of origin*: Australia
- *Description of scale*: Twenty items on a five-point Likert-form scale (Very low–Very high)
- *Developmental participants*: Not traced (n = 227)
- *Factors*: Four: (personal; communal; environmental; transcendental spiritual well-being)
- *Overall internal consistency*: Cronbach alpha 0.81–0.91

Example: Fisher and Brumley (2007) investigated the spiritual well-being of nurses (n = 212) and pastoral carers (n = 15) in relation to their workplace. It was found that nurses and pastoral carers who were more fulfilled in their relationships with themselves, others, the environment and/or God, reported that clients in hospitals and hospices received greater help in these dimensions from the services provided in their workplace. This indicates that the healthcare professionals' lived experience of spirituality may influence their perceptions of help provided to clients, aimed at nurturing their spiritual well-being. Thus, personal spirituality appears to contribute towards care as perceived by the nurses and pastoral carers.

5. Functional Assessment of Chronic Illness Therapy Spirituality Well-being Subscale (FACIT-SP) (Peterman *et al*, 2002)

- *Country of origin*: USA
- *Description of scale*: Twelve items on a five-point Likert-form scale (Not at all–Very much)
- *Developmental participants*: Cancer patients, psychotherapists, religious/spiritual experts (n = 200)
- *Factors*: Two (meaning/peace; faith)
- *Overall internal consistency*: Cronbach alpha 0.87

Example: Kinney *et al.* (2003) assessed the impact of an integrated mind–body–spirit self-empowerment programme for breast cancer survivors (n = 51) in a support-group format. Pre- and post-programme findings indicated a significant improvement in the participants' self-assessments of health and well-being on all measures including spiritual well-being. This improvement may be due to the beneficial effect of the support group and the self-empowerment techniques of the programme which appear to help them find meaning and purpose in life by utilising internal and external spiritual resources. Thus this underlines the importance of support groups and holistic interventions to patients with life-threatening illnesses.

Facet 3: Spiritual needs

An exploration of the different ways in which spiritual needs can be viewed has already been provided in Chapter 3. Two measures are presented in this section offering insights into what individuals may consider to be spiritual needs and how these spiritual needs may be addressed and supported by practitioners.

1. Spiritual Needs Inventory (SNI) (Hermann, 2006)

- *Country of origin*: USA
- *Description of scale*: Seventeen items on a Likert-form scale (Never–Always)
- *Developmental participants*: Hospice patients (n = 100)
- *Factors*: Five (outlook; inspiration; spiritual activities; religion; community)
- *Overall internal consistency*: Cronbach alpha 0.85

Example: Hampton *et al.* (2008) investigated the spiritual needs and unmet needs of clients with advanced cancer (n = 90) on admission to hospice-home care in the USA. Differences were found in patients' perceived needs whereby being with their family was reported by 80 per cent while prayer was identified by 50 per cent. Additionally, the most frequently reported unmet need was attending religious services. It implies that social support and religious support may assist patients to live harmoniously at the end of their life.

2. Spiritual Health Inventory (SHI) (Highfield, 1992)

- *Country of origin*: USA
- *Description of scale*: Thirty-one items on a five-point Likert-form scale (All the time–Never)
- *Developmental participants*: Oncology patients (n = 23) and their nurses (n = 27)
- *Factors*: Three (self-acceptance; relationships; hope)
- *Overall internal consistency*: Cronbach alpha 0.89 (patients) and 0.92 (nurses)

Example: Highfield (1992) explored the assessment of spiritual needs of patients as perceived by patients with cancer (n = 23) and their respective oncology nurse (n = 27). Spiritual health was defined as meeting the patients' spiritual needs of self-acceptance, relationships and hope. It was found that nurses inaccurately assessed their patients' spiritual health. Patients reported a high level of spiritual health with a positive relationship to age. Therefore the older ones were more likely to report higher spiritual health. While taking into consideration the complexity of assessing spiritual needs of patients (McSherry and Ross, 2002), the findings indicate the need to improve nurse–patient communication, while bracketing the assessors' personal experiences, in order to identify the actual spiritual needs of patients.

Facet 4: Meaning and purpose in life

In order to gain an understanding about the way in which meaning and purpose relate to spirituality, please refer to Chapters 2 and 3 (on 'a generic approach' and 'meaning and purpose' respectively). This section outlines four measures, which reveal that spirituality concerns the way in which individuals derive meaning, purpose, fulfilment and satisfaction from different aspects of life.

1. The Purpose In Life test (PIL) (Greenstein and Breibart, 2000)

- *Country of origin*: USA
- *Description of scale*: Twenty items on a seven-point bipolar Likert-form scale (categories not given)
- *Developmental participants*: Patients with cancer (n = 97)
- *Factors*: Two (meaning; purpose in life)
- *Overall internal consistency*: Cronbach alpha 0.90

Examples: Litwinczuk and Groh (2007) investigated the relationship between spirituality and purpose in life in a sample of clients with HIV infection (n = 46). Spirituality was found significantly correlated with purpose in life. Thus, when individuals manage to find purpose in life, they are more likely to have high scores of inner strength to cope with their HIV. This is supported by Cunningham (2005) who evaluated a psycho-educational-spiritual course on patients with various types and stages of cancer (n = 97). As the course progressed, the majority reported a greater ability to accept their situation, appreciated their daily life events more, had less conflict with others, and an enhanced sense of meaning in their lives. Therefore, addressing the spiritual dimension in the care of patients with terminal illnesses such as HIV and cancer may enhance their quality of life.

2. Personal meaning index (as part of Life Attitude Profile-Revised (LAP-R) (Reker, 1992)

- *Country of origin*: USA
- *Description of scale*: Items not given. Seven-point Likert-form scale (Very strongly disagree–Very strongly agree)
- *Developmental participants*: Derived from a literature review
- *Factors*: Three (zest for life; fulfilment; satisfaction)
- *Overall internal consistency*: Cronbach alpha 0.83

Example: Bauer-Wu and Farran (2005) compared meaning in life, spirituality, perceived stress and psychological distress between breast cancer survivors (n = 39) and healthy women (n = 39), all aged between 35 and 55 years. The cancer survivors without children were found to have less meaningful lives and greater stress than those with children and those in the healthy group. A positive significant correlation was found between meaning in life and spirituality. Conversely, a negative significant relationship was found between meaning in life and stress. This infers that living a meaningful life and connectedness with a higher power may yield lower levels of stress, and parallels the findings of Evangelista *et al.* (2003) who found a negative significant relationship between meaning and anxiety/depression and purpose in life. The majority of women were able to use coping strategies to help them regain control over their lives. Thus health professionals need to address meaning and purpose in life in their counselling and clinical care in order to help them cope with patients' ailments.

3. Spiritual Meaning Scale (SMS) (Mascaro *et al.*, 2004)

- *Country of origin*: USA
- *Description of scale*: Fourteen items on a five-point Likert-form scale (Totally disagree–Totally agree)
- *Developmental participants*: Students (n = 462)
- *Factors*: One (personal meaning)
- *Overall internal consistency*: Cronbach alpha 0.89

Example: Mascaro *et al.* (2004) conducted a correlational study on undergraduate students (n = 465), undertaking introductory psychology courses (females n = 215; males n = 247) with a mean age of 19.12 years. Findings identified a positive significant relationship between spiritual meaning and hope, while a negative significant correlation was found between spiritual meaning and depression, anxiety and antisocial features. Therefore, individuals who manage to find spiritual meaning in life are more likely to have less stress.

4. The meaning and purpose at work (Ashmos and Duchon, 2007)

- *Country of origin*: USA
- *Description of scale*: Thirty-four items on a five-point Likert-form scale (Excellent–Poor)
- *Developmental participants*: Health professions (n = 696)
- *Factors*: Five (sense of community; community at work; inner life; work unit community; work unit and meaningful work)
- *Overall internal consistency*: Cronbach alpha 0.857–0.914

Example: Ashmos and Duchon (2007) investigated the relationship of 696 health professionals' spirituality in six work units and patients' evaluation of the overall quality of care and evaluation of the overall sensitivity of the staff providing the care. It was found that the highest-performing unit has higher spirituality scores than the lowest-performing unit. A positive significant relationship was found between spirituality and work unit performance scores. This indicates that work unit performance may be greater in work units that foster a spiritual (spirit-friendly) climate, which may enable the workers' sense of meaningful work and their communal spirit at work.

Facet 5: Spiritual coping

Spiritual coping explores the way in which spirituality may assist individuals in coping with life events. Two measures are included in this section.

1. Spiritual Coping Strategies (SCS) scale (Baldacchino, 2002; Baldacchino and Buhagiar, 2003)

- *Country of origin*: Malta, Europe
- *Description of scale*: Twenty items on a four-point Likert-form scale (Use–Frequent use)
- *Developmental participants*: Nursing students (n = 55) and patients with myocardial infarction (n = 70)
- *Factors*: Two (religious spiritual coping strategies; non-religious spiritual coping strategies)
- *Overall internal consistency*: Cronbach alpha 0.82 (students) and 0.88 (patients)

Example: Baldacchino (2002) conducted a longitudinal study to identify relationships between spiritual coping and spiritual well-being, anxiety and depression of patients with first acute myocardial infarction (n = 70), aged 40–89 years (males n = 46; females n = 24). The findings showed a consistent increase in spiritual coping (both religious and non-religious) across time. Those patients who started off with extreme low scores in hospital kept their increased scores by the third month after discharge. Spiritual coping was positively significant with respect to spiritual well-being and inversely significant with respect to anxiety and depression across time. This implies the need to facilitate spiritual coping in hospitals and in the community as spiritual coping may be a resource of strength and power to individuals with a life-threatening illness (Otto, 1950).

2. The Spirituality and Chronic Pain Survey (SCPS) (Glover-Graf et al., 2007)

- *Country of origin*: USA
- *Description of scale*: Thirty-one items on a five-point Likert-form scale (Always–Never)
- *Developmental participants*: Patients with chronic pain (n = 95)
- *Factors*: Four (spiritual connection and meaning; spiritual

increase and hopefulness; spiritual decrease and punishment; spiritual power)

- *Overall internal consistency*: Cronbach alpha 0.89

Example: Glover-Graf *et al.* (2007) investigated spiritual and religious beliefs and practices among 95 patients receiving medical and psychological services for chronic pain (females n = 65; males n = 30) aged 24–86 years. The majority of patients perceived God/spiritual power as a resource of help, happiness, connection and meaning in life. Consequently, the most frequent coping strategy used was prayer (61 per cent). This indicates the importance of spiritual assessment in order to facilitate coping strategies in the process of dealing with pain.

Facet 6: Spirituality as part of quality of life

Within the healthcare literature there is a growing awareness of the impact that spirituality may have on an individual's quality of life. This work is being led mainly by the WHO.

1. World Health Organization Quality Of Life Spirituality Religiousness and Personal Beliefs (WHO-QOL SRPB) questionnaire (WHO-QOL Group, 2006)

- *Country of origin*: World Health Organization International Group Switzerland
- *Description of scale*: Thirty-two items on a Likert-form scale (not identified)
- *Developmental participants*: Healthy clients and patients with diverse religions (n = 5087)
- *Factors*: Eight (connectedness to a spiritual being or force; meaning in life; awe; wholeness and integration; spiritual strength; inner peace/serenity/harmony; hope and optimism; faith)
- *Overall internal consistency*: Cronbach alpha 0.91

Examples: The WHO-QOL SRPB Group (2006) conducted an international study in eighteen countries on various groups of healthy individuals and patients (n = 5087) with illness and a mean age of 41.3 years (males n = 2488; females n = 2599). The findings showed that healthy individuals were significantly more hopeful, with greater spirituality but with lower levels of religious faith. Women reported greater feelings of spiritual connection and religious faith than men. Those with less education reported greater religious faith but were less hopeful. In contrast, those with the highest education reported greater levels of hope and optimism. This is supported by Giovagnoli *et al.* (2006) who found significant relationship between spirituality and quality of life in patients with focal epilepsy (n = 32). Thus, spirituality needs to be addressed in patient care. Boero *et al.* (2005) assessed the spiritual dimension of quality of life of 116 health professionals (nurses n = 104; physicians n = 12) from three rehabilitation hospitals. Those who reported better clinical conditions showed higher spiritual quality of life. Those who reported good health scored higher in spirituality. Similarly, those who considered themselves religious and those reporting strong personal beliefs showed higher scores in quality of life. This implies that spirituality may have the potential to improve quality of life. Health professionals should consider the importance of addressing the patients' spiritual needs in order to help them enhance their quality of life.

Facet 7: Spiritual care

Spiritual care is defined as 'the activities and ways of being that bring spiritual quality of life, well-being and function' (Taylor, 2002, p. 24). This is consistent with literature which asserts that spiritual care is about being rather than doing (Bradshaw, 1994; Halm *et al.*, 2000). Thus, it is the heart and spirit by which care is delivered that may contribute to effective spiritual care. This section outlines four measure to offer insight into how spiritual care may be provided and the impact that such care may have on the patient experience.

1. Nurse's Role in Spiritual Care (NRSC) questionnaire
(Baldacchino, 2003)

- *Country of origin*: Malta, Europe
- *Description of scale*: Twenty-five items on a five-point Likert-form scale (Strongly agree–Strongly disagree)
- *Developmental participants*: Nursing students (n = 71)
- *Factors*: Three (facilitation of spiritual coping methods; promotion of interpersonal relationships, self-transcendence and achievement of life goals; enhancing nurse-patient communication and relief of spiritual distress)
- *Overall internal consistency*: Cronbach alpha 0.82

Example: Baldacchino (2003) investigated spiritual care as perceived by 53 patients with their first myocardial infarction (34 males; 19 females), aged 40–89 years; qualified nurses (n = 174) and nursing students (final year n = 178 and first year n = 90) and chaplains (n = 71). A discrepancy was found between health professionals and patients whereby qualified nurses agreed about the nurses' role in the spiritual dimension in care, with respect to factors like respecting patients' personal spiritual/religious objects, and allowing time for the patient to discuss his or her concerns and worries. However, the majority were uncertain about their role in patients' religious practices on the ward, such as facilitating private or group prayers, assisting patients in reading spiritual inspirational material, or praying for and/or with patients. This implies the need to address the patient's needs holistically by liaising with the interdisciplinary team, including the chaplain.

2. Spirituality and Spiritual Care Rating Scale (SSCRS)
(McSherry, 1997; McSherry *et al.*, 2002)

- *Country of origin*: United Kingdom
- *Description of scale*: Seventeen items on a five-point Likert-form scale (Strongly disagree–Strongly agree)
- *Developmental participants*: Nurses (n = 559)
- *Factors*: Four (existential search; rudiments of spiritual care; universality; individuality)
- *Overall internal consistency*: Cronbach alpha 0.64

Example: McSherry (1997) explored 559 nurses' perceptions of the concepts of spirituality and spiritual care. While considering these two concepts as very broad and subjective, nurses identified listening to and observing patients as the most frequent methods of assessing spiritual needs. Few nurses identified patients' spiritual needs through handover from other nurses, which may indicate an ethical dilemma to maintain confidentiality about personal spiritual issues (McSherry and Ross, 2002). Barriers to the delivery of spiritual care were: lack of human and other resources; lack of knowledge and confidence to address patients' spiritual needs; fear of mismanagement of spiritual needs; ambiguous definitions of spirituality and spiritual care; considering spiritual needs as too personal; and lack of privacy on the ward to address patients' needs. While considering these barriers, nurses emphasised the interdisciplinary team approach to help patients meet their needs.

3. The Treatment Spirituality/Religiosity Scale (TSRS)

(Lilies *et al.* 2008)

- *Country of origin*: USA
- *Description of scale*: Ten items; nominal data (True/False)
- *Developmental participants*: Patients with substance abuse disorder (n = 3018) and staff members (n = 329)
- *Factors*: One (spirituality/religiosity)
- *Overall internal consistency*: Cronbach alpha 0.77 (patients) and 0.83 (staff)

Example: Lilies *et al.* (2008) evaluated a new measure of spirituality/religiosity in the rehabilitation treatment of 3018 patients with substance abuse disorder. The TSRS could be completed by both patients and staff in order to detect the extent to which spirituality is integrated in care. Differences were identified in the degree of implementing spiritual/religious care in various treatment environments, which may be due to the positive outcome derived from the involvement of self-help groups in the rehabilitation process. Since TSRS may be used by both patients and health professionals, concurrent feedback from both patients and staff is possible, which may enhance the spiritual orientation to care.

4. Psychosocial Interventions for Existential Suffering questionnaire (Hirai *et al.* 2003)

- *Country of origin*: Japan
- *Description of scale*: Six items; (scale not given)
- *Developmental participants*: Psychiatrists (n = 146), psychologists (n = 42) and palliative care nurses (n = 268)
- *Factors*: Six (meaning-centred approach; providing comfortable environments; supportive–expressive approach; religious approach; education and coping skill training; being)
- *Overall internal consistency*: Cronbach alpha not given

Example: Hirai *et al.* (2003) investigated psychosocial interventions in palliative care in Japan for existential suffering. The effectiveness of these interventions for specific existential distress in the given vignettes was appraised by various healthcare professionals, namely 146 psychiatrists, 42 psychologists and 268 palliative care nurses. A supportive expressive approach was reported consistently by all three groups. Psychiatrists estimated the effectiveness of psycho-pharmacological treatment significantly higher than the psychologists and nurses. Conversely, nurses considered efficacy of all other interventions significantly higher than the psychiatrists and psychologists. Therefore an interdisciplinary team approach may relieve existential suffering in patients with terminal cancer.

Conclusion

While considering the complexity of the concepts of spirituality, spiritual well-being and spiritual care, the selection of the most appropriate tool or tools should be undertaken with caution in order to address the specific aims and objectives of the research study. On analysing the literature on development of new tools, some limitations were identified that restrict the reliability of the tool, such as recruitment of non-probability sampling technique, the use of cross-sectional designs that restrict collection of data at one point in time, and the lack of cross-cultural research, which inhibits the applicability of the tool to other cultures. For example, the majority of measures presented in this chapter originate from within the USA. Cross-cultural research demands rigorous translation of tools and checks of the appropriateness of the tool according to the character-istics of the sample recruited (Baldacchino and Buhagiar, 2003).

The absence of statistical power analysis which is a function of three other parameters (the significance level, sample size and effect size) may render the risk of committing a type I error and/or a type II error (Cohen, 1992; Martin and Thompson, 2000). A type I error is when an alternative hypothesis (H1) is falsely accepted, by wrongly rejecting a true null hypothesis (H0). Conversely, a type II error is when a false null hypothesis is accepted, by wrongly rejecting the research hypothesis (H1) that a relationship between variables exists (Polit and Sherman, 1990). The use of quantitative research renders the study more objective. However, since spirituality is highly subjective, it is recommended that mixed-method approaches are implemented in order to provide a rationale for the findings derived from the quantitative approach.

Spirituality may or may not consist of religiosity. Most of the tools are oriented towards Christianity. Thus, heterogeneous sampling techniques recruiting individuals with diverse religious affiliations, including atheists, may provide insight into the broad definition of spirituality. Despite the fact that a number of research tools have been developed, no single tool consists of all indicators of spirituality or spiritual care. This is because spirituality, spiritual well-being and spiritual needs are complex multidimensional concepts. Therefore, triangulation is recommended by the use of various research tools and additional investigators in order to obtain convergent validity in the data. While appreciating the diligence of the researchers who develop new tools in an attempt to further explore the concepts of spirituality, spiritual well-being and spiritual care, further psychometric testing of such tools is recommended in order to refine the indicators that may contribute towards reliability and validity of the overall research findings.

References

Arevalo S., Prado, G.M. and Amaro, H. (2008). 'Spirituality, sense of coherence, and coping responses in women receiving treatment for alcohol and drug addiction'. *Evaluation and Program Planning* 31, 113–23.

Ashmos, D. and Duchon, D. (2007). 'Nurturing the spirit at work: Impact on work unit performance'. *The Leadership Quarterly*, 16, 807–833.

Baldacchino, D. (2002). *Spiritual coping strategies, anxiety, depression and spiritual well-being of Maltese patients with first myocardial infarction: A longitudinal study.* PhD thesis. University of Hull.

Baldacchino, D. (2003). *Spirituality in Illness and Care.* Malta: Veritas Press.

Baldacchino, D. and Buhagiar, A. (2003). 'Psychometric evaluation of the Spiritual Coping Strategies scale in English, Maltese, back-translation and bilingual versions'. *Journal of Advanced Nursing*, 42(6), 558–70.

Bauer-Wu, F. and Farran, F. (2005). 'Meaning in life and psycho–spiritual functioning'. *Journal of Holistic Nursing*, 23(2), 172–90.

Boero, M.E., Caviglia M.L., Monteverdi, R., *et al.* (2005). 'Spirituality of health workers: A descriptive study'. *International Journal of Nursing Studies*, 42, 915–21.

Bradshaw, A. (1994). *Lighting the Lamp. The Spiritual Dimension of Nursing Care.* Middlesex: Scutari Press.

Burnard, P. and Morrison, D. (1994). *Nursing Research in Action: Developing Basic Skills*, 2nd edn. London: Macmillan.

Cohen, J. (1992). 'A power primer'. *Psychological Bulletin*, 112(1), 155–59.

Cunningham, A.J. (2005). 'Integrating spirituality into a group psychological therapy programme for cancer patients'. *Integrative Cancer Therapies*, 4(2), 178–86.

Evangelista, L.S., Doering, L. and Dracup, K. (2003). 'Meaning and life purpose: The perspectives of post-transplant women'. *Heart and Lung*, 32(4), 250–57.

Fetzer Group and National Institute on Ageing Working Group (1999). 'Brief multidimensional measure of religiousness/spirituality (BMMRS) for use in healthcare research'. Cited in: Rippentrop, A.E., Altmaier, E.M., Chen, J.J., *et al.* (2005). 'The relationship between religion/spirituality and physical health, mental health, and pain in a chronic pain population'. *Pain* 116, 311–21.

Fisher, J. (1999). 'Developing a spiritual health and life-orientation measure for secondary school students'. In: *Proceedings of University of Ballarat Annual Research Conference, 15 October 1999*. Victoria, Australia; University of Ballarat, pp. 57–63.

Fisher, J. and Brumley, D. (2007). 'Nurses' and carers' spiritual well-being in the workplace'. *Australian Journal of Advanced Nursing*, 25(4), 49–57.

Frankl, V.E. (1962). *Man's Search for Meaning: An Introduction to Logotherapy*. New York: Simon and Schuster.

Galanter, M., Dermatis, H., Bunt, G., Williams, C., Trujillo, M. and Steinke, P. (2007). 'Assessment of spirituality and its relevance to addiction treatment'. *Journal of Substance Abuse Treatment*, 33, 257–64.

Giovagnoli, A.R., Meneses, R.F. and Martins da Silva, A. (2006). 'The contribution of spirituality to quality of life in focal epilepsy'. *Epilepsy and Behaviour*, 9, 133–39.

Glover-Graf, N.M., Marini, I., Baker, J. and Buck, T. (2007). 'Religious and spiritual beliefs and practices of persons with chronic pain'. *Rehabilitation Counseling Bulletin*, 51(1), 21–33.

Greenstein, M. and Breitbart, W. (2000). 'Cancer and the experience of meaning: A group psychotherapy programme for people with cancer'. *American Journal of Psychotherapy*, 54, 486–500.

Halm, M.A., Myers, R.N. and Bennetts, P. (2000). 'Providing spiritual care to cardiac patients: Assessment and implications for practice'. *Critical Care Nurse*, 20(4), 54–72.

Hampton, D.M., Hollis, D.E., Lloyd, D.A., Taylor, J. and McMillan, S.C. (2008). 'Spiritual needs of persons with advanced cancer'. *American Journal of Hospice and Palliative Medicine*, 24(1), 42–48.

Hatch, R.L., Burg, M.A., Naberhaus, D.S. and Hellmich, L.K. (1998). 'The Spiritual Involvement and Beliefs Scale: Development and testing of a new instrument'. *Journal of Family Practice*, 46, 476–86.

Hermann, C.P. (2006). 'Development and testing of the spiritual needs inventory for patients near the end of life'. *Oncology Nursing Forum*, 33, 729–35.

Highfield, M.F. (1992). 'Spiritual health of oncology patients. Nurse and patient perspectives'. *Cancer Nursing*, 15(1), 1–8.

Hirai, K., Morita, T. and Kashiwagi, T. (2003). 'Professionally perceived effectiveness of psychosocial interventions for existential suffering of terminally ill cancer patients'. *Palliative Medicine*, 17, 688–94.

Holt, C., Clark,, E.M. and Klem, P.R. (2007). 'Expansion and validation of the spiritual locus of control scale'. *Journal of Health Psychology*, 12(4), 597–612.

Howden, J.W. (1992). 'Development and psychometric characteristics of the spirituality assessment scale. Doctoral dissertation, Texas Woman's University'. *Dissertation Abstracts International*, 54(1-B), 166B, UMI No. 9312917.

Hungelmann, J.A., Kenkel-Rossi,, E., Klassen, L. and Stollenwerk, R.M. (1985).

'Spiritual well-being in older adults: harmonious interconnectedness'. *Journal of Religion and Health*, 24(2), 147–53.

Hungelmann, J.A., Kenkel-Rossi, E., Klassen, L. and Stollenwerk, R.M. (1989). 'Development of the JAREL spiritual well-being scale'. In: *Classification of Nursing Diagnoses. Proceedings of the 8th Conference North American Nursing Diagnosis Association*. Philadelphia: JB Lippincott.

Jim, H.S., Purnell, J.Q. Richardson, S.A., Golden-Kreutz, D. and Anderson, B.L. (2006). 'Measuring meaning in life following cancer'. *Quality Life Research*, 15, 1355–71.

Kass, J., Firedman, R., Leserman, J., Zuttermeister, P. and Benson, H. (1991). 'Health outcomes and a new measure of spiritual experience'. *Journal for the Scientific Study of Religion*, 30, 203–11.

Kim, Y. and Seidlitz, L. (2002). 'Spirituality moderates the effect of stress on emotional and physical adjustment'. *Personality and Individual Differences*, 32, 1377–90.

Kinney, C.K., Rodgers, D.M., Nash, K.A. and Bray, C.O. (2003). 'Holistic healing for women with breast cancer through a mind, body and spirit self-empowerment programme'. *Journal of Holistic Nursing*, 21(3), 260–79.

Koenig, H.G., Larson, D.B. and Larson, S.S. (2001). 'Religion and coping with serious medical illness'. *Annals of Pharmacotherapy*, 35, 352–59.

Lilies, J., Gifford,, E., Humphreys, K. and Moos, R. (2008). 'Assessing spirituality/religiosity in the treatment environment: The treatment spirituality/religiosity scale'. *Journal of Substance Abuse Treatment*, 35(4), 1–7.

Litwinczuk, K.M. and Groh, C.J. (2007). 'The relationship between spirituality, purpose in life, and well-being in HIV-positive persons'. *Journal of the Association of Nurses in Aids Care*, 18(3), 13–22.

MacDonald, D.A. (2000). 'Spirituality: description, measurement and relation to the five factor model of personality'. *Journal of Personality*, 68(1). 153–97.

MacDonald, D.A. and Holland, D. (2002). 'Spirituality and boredom proneness'. *Personality and Individual Differences*, 32, 1113–19.

Martin, C.R. and Thompson, D.R. (2000). *Designing and Analysis of Clinical Nursing Research Studies*. London: Routledge.

Mascaro, N., Rosen, D.H. and Morey, L.C. (2004). 'The development, construct validity, and clinical utility of the spiritual meaning scale'. *Personality and Individual Differences*, 37, 845–60.

McClain-Jacobson, C., Rosenfield, B., Kosinski, A., Pessin, H., Cimino, J.E. and Breitbart, W. (2004). 'Belief in an afterlife, spiritual well-being and end-of-life despair in patients with advanced cancer'. *General Hospital Psychiatry*, 26, 484–86.

McSherry, W. and Ross, L. (2002). 'Dilemmas of spiritual assessment: considerations for nursing practice'. *Journal of Advanced Nursing*, 38(5), 479–88.

McSherry, W., Cash, K. and Ross, L. (2004). 'Meaning of spirituality: implications for nursing practice'. *Journal of Clinical Practice*, 13, 934–41.

McSherry, W., Draper, P. and Kendrick, D. (2002). 'Construct validity of a rating scale designed to assess spirituality and spiritual care'. *International Journal of Nursing Studies*, 39(7). 723–34.

McSherry, W. (1997). *A descriptive survey of nurses' perceptions of spirituality and spiritual care*. MPhil thesis. University of Hull.

Moberg, D.O. (1979). 'The development of social indicators of spiritual well-being for quality of life research'. In: D.O. Mober (ed.) *Spiritual Well-Being. Sociological Perspectives*. Washington: University Press of America, pp. 1–14.

Otto, R. (1950). *The Idea of the Holy: An Inquiry into the Non-Rational Factor in the Idea of the Divine and its Relation to the Rational*. London: Oxford University Press.

Paloutzian, R.F. and Ellison, C.W. (1991). *Manual for Spiritual Well-Being*. Nyack, NY: Life Advance.

Peterman, A.H., Fitchett, G., Brady, M.J., Hernandez, L. and Cella, D. (2002). 'Measuring spiritual well-being in people with cancer: The functional assessment of chronic illness therapy–Spiritual Well-being Scale (FACIT-Sp-Ex)'. *Annals of Behavioural Medicine*, **24**, 49–58.

Polit, D.F. and Beck, C.T. (2006). *Essentials of Nursing Research: Methods, Appraisal and Utilization*, 6th edn. Philadelphia: Lippincott Company.

Polit, D.F. and Hungler, B. (1999). *Nursing Research: Principles and Methods*, 5th edn. Philadelphia: JB Lippincott.

Polit, F.P. and Sherman, R.E. (1990). 'Statistical power in nursing research'. *Nursing Research*, **39**(6), 365–69.

Reker, G.T. (1992). *Life Attitude Profile* (Revised Manual). Ontario, Canada: Student Psychologists.

Rippentrop, A.E., Altmaier, E.M., Chen, J.J., Found, E.M. and Keffala, V.J. (2005). 'The relationship between religion/spirituality and physical health, mental health, and pain in a chronic pain population. *Pain*, **116**, 311–21.

Rotter, J.B. (1966) 'Generalised expectancies for internal versus external control of reinforcement'. In: J.B. Rotter (ed.) *Social Learning and Clinical Psychology*. Englewood Cliffs, NJ: Prentice Hall.

Seidlitz, L., Abernethy, A.D., Duberstein, P.R., Evinger, J.S., Chang, T.H. and Lewis, B. (2002). 'Development of the spiritual transcendence index'. *Journal for the Scientific Study of Religion*, **41**(3), 439–53.

Swinton, J. and Narayanasamy, A. (2002). 'A critical view of spirituality and spiritual assessment by P. Draper and W. McSherry'. *Journal of Advanced Nursing*, **40**(2), 158–60.

Taylor, E.J. (2002). *Spiritual Care. Nursing Theory, Research and Practice*. Upper Saddle River, New York: Prentice Hall.

Taylor, E.J. (2006). 'Prevalence and associated factors of spiritual needs among patients with cancer and family caregivers'. *Oncology Nursing Forum*, **33**, 729–35.

Witt Sherman, D., Ye X., McSherry, C., Calabrese, M., Parkas, V. and Gatto, M. (2005). 'Spiritual well-being as a dimension of quality of life for patients with advanced cancer and AIDS and their family caregivers: Results of a longitudinal study'. *American Journal of Hospice and Palliative Medicine*, **22**(5), 349–62.

World Health Organization WHO-QOL SRPB Group (2006). 'A cross-cultural study of spirituality, religion and personal beliefs as components of quality of life'. *Social Studies and Medicine*, **62**, 1486–97.

Chapter 7
Assessing and improving the quality of spiritual care
Mark Cobb

Introduction

Spiritual assessment is the focus of much discussion and debate within healthcare because it is often considered crucial in ensuring that patients receive the spiritual care that they need. Quality of care is said to be achieved when patients receive the treatment and support they need, so we need to find ways of evaluating whether spiritual care is of sufficient quality to benefit patients. As we shall see this is a more complex question than it first appears, because both quality and spirituality are terms that have a range of meanings and interpretations. But what is clear is that quality defines a significant part of the healthcare agenda and spirituality is implicated in it through disparate policy statements, standards of care, statements of professional competence and evaluations of the performance of services.

In what follows we shall consider the nature of the current quality agenda and identify which elements of quality have a relationship with spiritual care from the aspirational level of policy to the practitioner level of competencies. We shall then review how the quality of spiritual care can be assessed using the widely used method of clinical audit, and differentiate the measurement of outcomes for the purposes of research from the evaluation of practice for audit. What will become clear is that audit alone is an inadequate process for quality improvement, and we shall explore some ideas about the gaps between our knowledge of spirituality in healthcare and the way this knowledge is implemented in practice. Spiritual assessment tools therefore come to be seen as 'knowledge products' that depend upon an implementation process to enable them to be successfully used in practice. Finally, we shall consider an example of a collaborative model of quality improvement that aims to bridge the gap between what we *know* and what we *do* and apply it to spiritual care.

The quality agenda

The quality agenda

Quality has become a common qualifier in the way healthcare is described and promoted. High-quality treatment and care are rightly set as the goals for healthcare organisations and their workforce, and are motivated by ethical obligations, statutory responsibilities and the expectations of those who use healthcare services. By *quality* we simply mean that patients receive the care and treatment they need, but behind this definition there is a growing understanding that quality not only depends upon the way we care for people but also the way health services are organised, managed and planned. Quality therefore is something that relates to the whole system of care, with roles and responsibilities at all levels, and consequences for both individuals and populations. From this perspective of the health system the World Health Organization provides a working definition of quality healthcare that comprises six dimensions: effective, efficient, accessible, acceptable/patient-centred, equitable, and safe (World Health Organization, 2006).

Quality in this sense combines both a positive intention and a preventative constraint: on the one hand it is about consistently attaining good outcomes, through personalised care that is available to all in need; and on the other hand it is related to the avoidance of harm, the mitigation of errors, the reduction of wasteful processes, and the limitation of variances. These parameters of quality are found in many of the key documents of the National Health Service (NHS) and of the organisations that regulate it, scrutinise it, and evaluate its effectiveness (such as the Healthcare Commission who measure the performance of health services against standards and criteria of quality). One of the latest chapters in this agenda is the review of the NHS in England, led by Lord Darzi, which sets out some aspirations for further reform to deliver high-quality care which is described as 'care where patients are in control, have effective access to treatment, are safe, and where illnesses are not just treated, but prevented' (Department of Health, 2008a, p. 45). In particular Darzi emphasises the need to measure quality with comparable metrics that will help organisations review and improve the quality of their services and to make these available to the public in so-called 'quality accounts'.

Below these high-level definitions, quality has to be translated into practical and tangible terms that can be demonstrated, understood and achieved. This is where quality is often quantified in terms such as performance ratings, patient satisfaction scores, waiting-list targets and mortality rates; and once quantified it can be subjected to measurement, and the performance of staff, services and organisations can be subject to management. At this organisational level, quality may be expressed within best practice standards and guidelines that are service-specific (e.g. accident and emergency) or condition-specific (e.g. diabetes) and informed by summations of the best evidence from research. At an individual level, quality may be described in the form of competency frameworks which summarise the knowledge, skills, attitudes and behaviour practitioners are expected to attain through education and training, and to demonstrate in their practice. These explicit statements of quality can then be systematically monitored and evaluated, any shortfalls addressed and improvements verified, thus providing an indication of the levels of quality being achieved. One process that provides such a quality feedback loop is an audit cycle, which is a systematic means of evaluating aspects of healthcare against explicit outcomes.

Levels of quality

Levels of quality

Having set out the quality agenda we now need to ask what is meant by quality spiritual care? The criteria published by the independent regulator for health and social care services (Care Quality Commission, 2009) contain no explicit reference to spiritual care. However, there are general requirements about respecting diversity, preferences and choices (Domain 4) and about treating patients, relatives and carers with dignity and respect (core standard C13a). There is an echo of this in the Darzi review, which calls for services to be more responsive to individuals, whereby quality must be patient-centred so that it includes the patient's experience of care, meaning 'the compassion, dignity and respect with which patients are treated' (Department of Health, 2008a, p. 47). In addition, the Care Quality Commission states that patients have the right to have their religious dietary requirements met (C15b), to access health services equally (C18), and to have access to private areas to fulfil their religious and spiritual needs (C20b). These latter criteria relate to recently introduced legislative and regulatory equality frameworks which include unlawful discrimination on the grounds of religion or belief (Department of Health, 2009).

At the service level, the Department of Health have issued a best practice guide about the provision of 'spiritual care that is equal, just, humane and respectful' and where 'meeting the varied spiritual needs of patients, staff and visitors is fundamental to the care the NHS provides' (Department of Health, 2003, p. 5). The guidance addresses how to meet spiritual and religious needs through NHS chaplains and faith community representatives, and it has nothing further to say about other healthcare professions. Similarly NHS Scotland requires each of its Boards to develop a spiritual care policy to ensure the provision of spiritual care is responsive to patients' needs with adequately resourced 'spiritual care services', which again refers to chaplaincy (NHS Scotland, 2008a).

There are condition-specific guidelines which make reference to spiritual care. An example is the guidance commissioned by the National Institute for Health and Clinical Excellence (NICE) on dementia, which takes a person-centred approach relating to an individual's religious beliefs and spiritual identity. This is made explicit in a number of places, for instance, in relation to non-cognitive symptoms that cause distress or result in challenging behaviour. It recommends that people with dementia are offered a comprehensive assessment that includes 'individual biography, including religious beliefs and spiritual and cultural identity' (National Institute for Health and Clinical Excellence, 2007, p. 260). The most comprehensive inclusion of spiritual care is found in the NICE guidance on palliative and supportive care. This contains both key recommendations about meeting the spiritual needs of patients, with a whole chapter devoted to spiritual support services. In summary the recommendations establish that patients and their carers should have access to spiritual support that is an integral part of their health and social care, and should be 'open to similar levels of scrutiny and supervision as other aspects of non-physical care' (National Institute for Health and Clinical Excellence, 2004, p. 98). The English and Scottish strategies for end-of-life care both include access to spiritual care within their descriptions of high-quality care (Department of Health, 2008b; Scottish Government, 2008).

It is evident there is no extant blueprint for quality spiritual care that can be applied comprehensively throughout the healthcare services; however there are examples of quality being defined at some level in relation to specific aspects of care or to particular conditions. Finally, we need to consider whether we can define quality spiritual care at the level of practice. The NHS Knowledge and Skills Framework (KSF) describes the competencies needed by non-medical staff to deliver quality services. The framework acknowledges that health and well-being needs may be emotional, mental, physical, social, and spiritual. Consequently the assessment, planning and care of patients should include aspects of spiritual health and well-being through, for example, 'enabling people to take part in prayer and worship and other spiritual activities' (NHS, 2004, p. 107).

There are also profession-specific competencies which describe the practice required to deliver quality spiritual care. The professional associations of healthcare chaplains, for example, have adopted a comprehensive set of capabilities and competences that include the knowledge and skills for professional practice, assessment and intervention, institutional practice, and reflective practice (NHS, Scotland, 2008b). In professions where spiritual care at some level is one aspect of their role, these competencies are more succinct. For instance, the Royal College of Nursing has described a set of spiritual competencies they expect of advanced nurse practitioners (Royal College of Nursing, 2008, p. 19). They should:

- respect the inherent worth and dignity of each person and the right to express spiritual beliefs;

- assist patients and families to meet their spiritual needs in the context of health and illness experiences, including referral for pastoral services;

- assess the influence of patients' spirituality on their healthcare behaviours and practices;

- incorporate patients' spiritual beliefs in the care plan.

Spiritual care and its cognates are evident in many descriptions of quality healthcare from the aspirational national level to the competency level of the practitioner. In the practical process which translates this into reality an assessment of spiritual needs is widely recognised to be necessary. We should expect therefore that spiritual care in practice, and spiritual assessment in particular, should be subject to scrutiny in relation to its quality, and evaluated to ensure that it is meeting the needs of patients. We could go still further and ask whether spiritual care for patients is fulfilling the six dimensions of quality, by reviewing whether it is effective, efficient, accessible, patient-centred, equitable, and safe. This implies a need to determine whether practice is in accordance with guidance and fulfils the parameters of quality expected by patients, professionals and the healthcare regulators.

Clinical audit

Clinical audit

One of the most widely adopted methods for evaluating the quality of healthcare is that of clinical audit which has been described as 'a quality improvement process that seeks to improve patient care and outcomes through systematic review of care against explicit criteria and the implementation of change' (National Institute for Health and Clinical Excellence, 2002, p. 10). When considering the quality of spiritual care, an audit process provides the opportunity to think critically and carefully about how a philosophy of care should be implemented in practice and what might be the indicators of good spiritual care. An audit requires that a process of care is deconstructed for examination and typically three domains of care are distinguished: the structure or resources required; the process or practices implemented; and the outcome or the effects on the patient (Donabedian, 2005).

Describing what is meant by quality is pivotal to an audit and the use of valid criteria is no less important in the case of spiritual care. If standards are vague or unreliable then they will not enable a rigorous audit that can contribute to the assessment and improvement of quality. Standards and criteria are usually developed from a range of sources including clinical guidelines, user and practitioner consensus, and benchmarking between comparable services. Good practice (Moullin, 2002, p. 69) suggests that they should be:

- realistic and attainable within available resources
- based on the views of service users
- real and important indicators of quality
- expressed clearly and unambiguously
- consistent with service aims and values
- set with the people who will be asked to achieve them
- measurable and capable of being monitored.

The content and specificity of criteria are highly dependent upon what can be measured, particularly when devising outcome criteria, and this operational factor can be a significant limitation to the assessment of quality. In terms of spiritual care, more direct data is usually available for structure and process criteria. For example, the Healthcare Commission's review of acute inpatient mental health services includes a care records audit that asks: 'During the first seven days of admission, did the inpatient assessment of the service user's need record spiritual needs?' (Healthcare Commission, 2008a). This is a clear criterion and standard that can be easily measured from a review of patient records. However, their results (41.1 per cent 'Yes', 58.6 per cent 'No' and 0.3 per cent blanks) based on 3450 care records audited across 69 trusts, tell us little about the quality of the assessment, how it was translated into care (process) and the effect on patient health and well-being (outcome).

An example of a more systematic approach comes from the specialty of palliative care that has done more than most to translate its holistic philosophy into practice. In this case the audit of spiritual care is one element of a comprehensive audit package for palliative care developed by a multidisciplinary team that takes structure, process and outcome as its framework. The overall standard is that the spiritual needs of patients and carers are integrated into the assessment and delivery of palliative care, and this is measured against criteria in each of the domains of care, examples of which are given below (Hunt *et al.*, 2003).

Structural criteria

- The multidisciplinary team includes a chaplain who, as the spiritual care specialist, is responsible for coordinating religious and spiritual care.

- The multidisciplinary team has specific documentation for the recording of religious and spiritual care planning.

Process criteria

- The multidisciplinary team uses consistent assessment processes to inform the planning of spiritual care interventions.
- The multidisciplinary team review identifies which team member leads the intervention.

Outcome criteria

- The patient states that members of the multidisciplinary team have enabled the exploration of their beliefs and practices in the context of their illness.
- The multidisciplinary team records the impact of spiritual care on symptom management, psychological and social palliative care, including working with carers.

As this example illustrates, an important source of data to assess outcome criteria is that of the patient or service user. This may be direct (e.g. patient interview) or indirect (e.g. case review), but involving patients in an audit needs a similar consideration to that of their participation in research in terms of ethical issues, methodology, inclusion criteria, the type of population sample, practical administration of the audit tool, and the analysis of the collected data.

Categorical and contingent criteria

Categorical and contingent criteria

What is evaluated as an outcome, and therefore what is measured or asked of patients, is highly dependent upon the operative construct of spiritual care. Specifically, what effects does spiritual care have upon patients that are accessible to an audit exercise? In addition, contextual factors are also an unavoidable determinant of spiritual assessments, and so is the evaluation of their use in practice. What might be possible in the multidisciplinary environment of specialist palliative care becomes less realistic in, say, an acute general surgery setting. The challenge therefore is to balance standards that should rightly be expected of healthcare in general (e.g. dignity) while recognising aspects of spiritual care that may be conditional upon the clinical setting, or the particular patient group, or the needs of individual patients.

One approach to addressing these factors is to develop categorical criteria that apply in general cases and contingent criteria that depend upon the context and the particular patient group or individual case. This enables levels of differentiation to be applied that recognise a first-stage general screening assessment and a subsequent (more thorough) assessment that may be required to identify and understand specific issues. For example the developers of the palliative care tool cited above recognise three levels of assessment: the categorical level is that of a routine assessment for all patients, and the contingent levels are more in-depth assessments indicated by complex issues that are presented by some – but not all – patients (Hunt *et al.*, 2003). However, assessment of spiritual needs may take a more biographical or narrative form where the content of the assessment is determined by the patient rather than a standardised interview tool. An example of this is the holistic common assessment for people with cancer which recommends that the process should be 'patient-concerns led' and helping patients to assess their own needs should be central to the process. The assessment should largely follow a 'conversational style' (Cancer Action Team, 2007, p. 5).

The holistic framework is divided into five domains, one of which concerns spiritual well-being and contains five items as shown in Box 7.1.

Box 7.1

Guidance and prompts for assessors from Domain 5 of the holistic framework (Cancer Action Team, 2007)

Item 5.1: Faith/belief

An introductory, exploratory question to determine the patient's existing faith/belief, be it 'religious' or non-religious, conventional or unconventional.

Item 5.2: Worries and challenges

Identify the person's worries related to spiritual well-being, and the challenges they perceive.

Impact of diagnosis or illness on faith.

Coping with impact of diagnosis.

Item 5.3: Needs related to spiritual well-being

Identify practical, support or other needs related to religion or spiritual matters.

Religious items (e.g. religious texts or books, prayer mat, religious objects, holy water)

Someone to speak to: faith leader or minister (e.g. minister, chaplain, vicar, priest, imam, rabbi, spiritual leader, church leader), or other person.

Help: things to help practice.

Prayer: prayer with other people or family.

Chapel; prayer room; space to pray; quiet room; privacy; private space; ablution.

Item 5.4: Restrictions related to culture or belief system

Practical, support or other restrictions related to person's cultural or ethnic background, or belief system.

Requirements; restrictions; diet; medicines; treatment products (e.g. blood products); transplantation.

Item 5.5: Life goals

A person's concerns or desires regarding a 'goal' they want to achieve in their life, such as attending a forthcoming wedding.

Important occasions; family gatherings; holidays; big events.

The recommended conversational approach to this form of assessment can be evaluated against relevant structure, process and outcome criteria through an audit process. In this case, structure criteria could include the competency of staff required to undertake the assessment and the use of documentation to record patient needs. Process criteria could describe the inclusion of this assessment within the patient pathway and the mechanisms for incorporating spiritual needs within care planning and clinical decision-making. Outcome criteria could include patients evaluating that they were receiving the spiritual and practical support they needed and that made them feel more able to cope with their illness.

Outcomes of spiritual care

Outcomes of spiritual care

Outcomes of care are important indicators of its effectiveness. They range from general satisfaction ratings of care and changes in health status, to narrowly defined physiological functions. Healthcare research typically investigates the nature of the relationship between a healthcare intervention and its outcome with the aim of identifying interventions that produce the most beneficial effects. For example, a review of randomised or quasi-randomised controlled trials of relaxation techniques with people who are depressed concluded that they 'were more effective at reducing self-rated depressive symptoms than no or minimal treatment. However, they were not as effective as psychological treatment'. This suggests that relaxation may be a useful first-line intervention (Jorm *et al.*, 2008). In audit there is an assumption, evidence-based where possible, that the intervention or process is related to good outcomes. Consequently, audit depends upon research to identify effective interventions and it may also provide evidence of the significance and relevance of topics to the quality of care, which in this case is spirituality.

There is a growing body of published research that aims to investigate the relationship of spirituality to health and to identify beneficial effects (Koenig *et al.*, 2001). These studies use measures of spirituality to describe religious and spiritual characteristics (e.g. the SpREUK questionnaire; Bussing *et al.*, 2007) and to measure spiritual well-being (e.g. the FACIT-Sp scale; Peterman *et al.*, 2002). It may be assumed that such measures have the potential to be adapted for the purpose of quality monitoring in healthcare, particularly in relationship to outcomes of spiritual care. Regardless of their validity and utility in research they can be problematic when applied to evaluating clinical practice. The context and purpose of research is very different to that of care, but more critically many measures do not differentiate sufficiently between spirituality and health outcomes. Koenig calls these 'contaminated measures' because they include positive experiences and psychological traits, and he comments that:

> *Since research findings have linked religious involvement to better health, health practices, and medical decision-making, it may be appropriate to include spirituality in discussions related to providing whole person healthcare. However, including religious or spiritual factors in measures of health itself (where health is an outcome to be studied) makes research between spirituality and health difficult to interpret for the same reasons that research using contaminated measures of spirituality is problematic.*

Koenig, 2008, p. 353

This is a cautionary note for measuring outcomes related to spirituality and again it highlights issues around the construct of factors being assessed. There are evident differences between the need to measure outcomes in research studies and the assessment of interventions as part of a quality management process. But both require reliable and valid methods, and spiritual assessment tools developed for healthcare practice need to be aware of the contamination with the positive traits that Koenig is critical of. When it comes to measuring outcome criteria in an audit it may be unrealistic to aim for the level of differentiation achieved in research, and more global and inclusive measures may be good enough for the practical purposes of understanding the impact of interventions with patients. The test is whether what is measured in audit is robust enough to indicate the quality of care provided. If it fails this test then healthcare services may not be able to demonstrate how consistently and at what level they are responding to the spiritual needs of their patients and, more importantly, patients may be failing to receive the care and support they require.

Finally, outcome measures relating to spiritual care go beyond the individual impact upon patients and its effectiveness for individuals. If we return to the six dimensions of quality described at the beginning of this chapter then it is possible to develop outcome criteria that can indicate a more comprehensive concept of quality. One approach could be to develop an audit tool across organisations based upon a common dataset that enables a comparative evaluation. This requires a consensus about standards of practice and the data required to measure them. Analysis of the results enables comparison with a peer group and identifies variations against the agreed best practice. An example of this is the National Care of the Dying Audit of Hospitals which is an audit across participating acute hospitals against the standards of care within the *Liverpool Care Pathway for the Dying Patient* (Ellershaw and Wilkinson, 2003). The audit has shown that the assessment of spiritual and religious needs took place in only half of cases and was often poorly documented (Marie Curie Palliative Care Institute Liverpool, 2009). While in this example the measures are limited to process criteria, further dimensions of quality could be assessed through a benchmarking-type audit, some examples of which are given below:

Effectiveness: Patient satisfaction with spiritual support provided.
Efficiency: Workforce levels within organisations and their activity levels in relation to overall admissions.

Accessibility: The availability of the service, response times to referrals and the provision of spiritual facilities.

Personalised: The provision of elements of care in relation to the needs of patient groups and communities (e.g. religious diets).

Equitable: Referral for spiritual care in relation to gender, age, ethnicity and primary diagnosis.

Safety: Levels of untoward and patient safety incidents relating to spiritual care.

Improving the quality of spiritual care

Improving the quality of care

Audit is a common quality initiative within the health services but it is not without its limitations. In relation to spiritual care, one of the major limitations is the extent to which a clear and practical model of it can be developed and then deconstructed into the component parts of structure, process and outcome required for the purposes of an audit. But looked at the other way round we also need to be asking if audit is a good method to frame the practice of spiritual care, evaluate its effectiveness and support improvement. In a review of randomised trials of audit and feedback the authors concluded that the evidence 'does not support mandatory use of audit and feedback as an intervention to change practice. However, audit is commonly used in the context of governance and it is essential to measure practice to know when efforts to change practice are needed' (Jamtvedt *et al.*, 2006). Audit therefore is a tool that can be used to indicate when we are failing to deliver effective spiritual care and when change is required, but we may need to consider other strategies to bring about the improvements that are required.

Øvretveit (2003) identified thirteen types of strategy reported in the research literature to improve quality in hospitals, concluding that there is no strong evidence of the effectiveness of any of them. This betrays a debate among researchers about methods for evaluating quality strategies and it raises some critical questions about how healthcare resources should be committed to support the quality agenda. It is unlikely that one method will deliver the many demands of quality improvement and it is a helpful reminder that the multidimensional nature of quality will require more than a one-dimensional approach. If we accept that clinical audit is a well-established process that can indicate shortcomings in the quality of spiritual care then what strategies might we use to improve spiritual care?

A starting place is recognising that there is a gap between the practice within healthcare services and the experiential and research knowledge evident in the literature. A good example is that the development of spiritual assessment tools has been insufficient to make a significant impact in routine practice. There is a translational gap here between the creation of knowledge of spiritual care and its practical application. Graham *et al.* (2006) provide a conceptual framework for understanding the process of knowledge translation which we can apply to spiritual care with some simplification. In this scheme there is a knowledge creation phase, followed by an action phase. Spiritual assessment tools can be classified as knowledge that has been synthesised, distilled and refined into a practical form that can be considered a knowledge product which is tailored to the needs of potential users. This interconnects with an action cycle involving the following phases (Graham *et al.*, 2006):

Adapting the identified knowledge or research to the local context.

Assessing barriers to using the knowledge.

Selecting, **tailoring** and **implementing** interventions to promote the use of knowledge (i.e. implementing the change).

Monitoring knowledge use.

Evaluating the outcomes of using the knowledge.

Sustaining ongoing knowledge use.

Translating knowledge of spiritual care into practical action requires going beyond dissemination to strategically planned implementation. It involves a chain of critical processes that are transacted across different stakeholders, with differing purposes and cultures. For example, a study to explore the ideas about quality held by hospital-based doctors and nurses in Geneva found that they focused on the technical and human aspects of care (knowledge and skills, personal motivation, and the ability and willingness to collaborate) and rarely mentioned clinical guidelines or dimensions of efficiency, safety and equity (Hudelson *et al.*, 2008). Similarly there will be different forms of knowledge that relate to spirituality and the practice of spiritual care, some of which will be highly experiential and personal and others which will be abstract and conceptual. Batalden and Davidoff (2007) propose that there is the knowledge derived from empirical (scientific) studies, knowledge of the particular context of care, knowledge of measuring improvement, knowledge of how to apply generalised evidence to the particular context, and knowledge required for making change happen. They say on the subject:

Acquiring these five kinds of knowledge requires both scientific and experiential learning. Reflection on the nature of these five knowledge systems, how they grow and change, and the ways in which they work together to move evidence into practice will be essential if we are going to learn about learning. Doing so will generate a kind of 'meta-knowledge' that will be essential over the long run in becoming progressively better at improvement.

Batalden and Davidoff, 2007, p. 2

Implementing knowledge that has the potential to improve the quality of spiritual care requires an understanding of the prevailing knowledge systems that influence stakeholders. Perhaps too much of the focus on spiritual care has been on the knowledge creation phase, with not enough on the application phase. However convincing the evidence and the arguments of the need for spiritual assessment, the practice will remain limited without an understanding of the barriers to its adoption across relevant stakeholders and how their knowledge enables or inhibits the translation of spiritual care concepts into practice. Equally, an understanding of how different stakeholders learn, and how practice within organisations and services can change, will be vital to make and sustain improvements.

Applying an improvement model

Issues of knowledge translation are addressed in a model of healthcare improvement that has been developed by the American Institute for Healthcare Improvement (IHI). Their model, known as the Breakthrough Series, aims to bridge the gap between what we know and what we do and recognises the limitations of the dissemination of knowledge and didactic educational methods such as lectures and conferences. The model is designed to support healthcare organisations through collaborative improvement and is founded on the following set of fundamental premises (Kilo, 1998):

- A substantial gap exists between knowledge and practice in healthcare.
- Broad variation in practice is pervasive.
- Examples of improved practices and outcomes exist, but they need to be described and disseminated to other organisations.
- Collaboration between professionals working towards clear aims enables improvement.
- Healthcare outcomes are the result of processes.
- Understanding the science of rapid cycle improvement can accelerate demonstrable improvement.

The Breakthrough Series was designed for collaboratives of between 20 and 40 organisations working together for up to 12 months on major clinical issues. However, the model offers some useful principles that can be applied to spiritual care, the most important of which is taking a systems approach to change. A faculty in the relevant discipline is recruited, with experts in the relevant subject matter as well as 'application experts'. Multidisciplinary teams from different organisations then apply to join a collaborative and learn from a process that includes face-to-face learning sessions and action periods in which teams test and implement changes in their local setting. A model for organising and implementing improvement through a cyclical process is taught to the participants and this facilitates successful changes through learning (Institute for Healthcare Improvement, 2003).

There are a number of key lessons from this model that can be applied to spiritual care. First, improving the spiritual care of patients must warrant sufficient interest, commitment and priority to generate the necessary momentum to drive an improvement process. Second, there must be a critical mass of experts in the subject, application experts and multidisciplinary organisational teams to form a collaborative within which to develop understanding, share knowledge, propose changes and identify measures of improvement. Third, participants must follow a systematic process to learn, test, implement and evaluate changes to spiritual care practice to support its success and sustainability.

The development of spiritual assessment tools and particular interventions to address spiritual needs will flounder without an understanding of the ways in which that knowledge is adopted and applied to practice within the context of healthcare organisations. Central to this is an awareness of the organisational barriers and resistance that can block beneficial change, such as lack of ownership and inadequate or inappropriate leadership, and how these difficulties can be overcome (Scott *et al.*, 2003). Consequently improvements to spiritual care are likely to remain local, incremental, *ad hoc* and disparate without a concerted focus and a systemic process of change. While such a model may seem antithetical to the highly personal world of spirituality and the interpersonal practice of spiritual care, it has the potential to provide a more robust and critical process for improving the structures, processes and outcomes of spiritual care in ways which can be applied across healthcare systems.

Conclusion

It is reasonable to suggest that the quality of spiritual care is related in part to the quality of spiritual assessment which serves the decisive function of identifying a patient's needs. This chapter has critically examined this process of care, and questioned what is meant by quality, the ways it is measured and how it might be improved. Significantly it has differentiated the role of audit in identifying practice that fails to meet agreed standards from strategies of improving practice. What has become clear is that improvements to the quality of spiritual care cannot be achieved simply by producing a spiritual assessment tool, for in itself this cannot bridge the knowledge practice gap. What is required is an understanding of the wider healthcare system, the way knowledge can be translated into processes and practices, and the barriers that may prevent necessary developments. This suggests the need for a more systematic and collaborative approach to improving spiritual care for patients that can provide the critical and credible mass for sustained and effective change.

References

Batalden, P.B. and Davidoff, F. (2007). 'What is 'quality improvement' and how can it transform healthcare?' *Quality and Safety in Healthcare*, **16**, 2–3.

Büssing, A., Ostermann, T. and Koenig, H. (2007). 'Relevance of religion and spirituality in German patients with chronic diseases'. *International Journal of Psychiatry in Medicine*, **37**(1), 39–57.

Cancer Action Team (2007). *Holistic Common Assessment of Supportive and Palliative Care Needs for Adults with Cancer: Assessment Guidance.* London: Cancer Action Team.

Care Quality Commission (2009). *Criteria for Assessing Core Standards in 2009/10: Acute Trusts.* London: Care Quality Commission.

Department of Health (2003). *NHS Chaplaincy: Meeting the Religious and Spiritual Needs of Patients and Staff.* London: Department of Health.

Department of Health (2008a). *High Quality Care for All: NHS Next Stage Review Final Report.* London: The Stationery Office.

Department of Health (2008b). *End of Life Care Strategy.* London: Department of Health.

Department of Health (2009). *Religion or Belief: A Practical Guide for the NHS.* London: Department of Health.

Donabedian, A. (2005). 'Evaluating the quality of medical care'. *The Milbank Quarterly*, **83**(4): 691–729.

Ellershaw, J. and Wilkinson, S. (2003). *Care of the Dying: A Pathway to Excellence.* Oxford: Oxford University Press.

Graham, I.D., Logan, J., Harrison, M.B., *et al.* (2006). 'Lost in knowledge translation: Time for a map?' *The Journal of Continuing Education in the Health Professions*, **26**(1), 13–24.

Healthcare Commission (2008a). *Acute Inpatient Mental Health Service Review Results of the Care Records Audit.* London: Healthcare Commission.

Healthcare Commission (2008b). *Criteria for Assessing Core Standards in, 2008/09: Acute Trusts.* London: Healthcare Commission.

Hudelson, P., Cleopas, A., Kolly, V., Chopard, P. and Perneger, T. (2008). 'What is quality and how is it achieved? Practitioners' views versus quality models'. *Quality and Safety in Healthcare*, **17**, 31–36.

Hunt, J., Cobb, M., Keeley, V.L. and Ahmedzai, S.H. (2003). The quality of spiritual care – Developing a standard. *International Journal of Palliative Nursing*, **9**(5), 208–15.

Institute for Healthcare Improvement (2003). *The Breakthrough Series: IHI's Collaborative Model for Achieving Breakthrough Improvement.* Boston: Institute for Healthcare Improvement.

Jamtvedt, G., Young, J.M., Kristoffersen, D.T., O'Brien, M.A. and Oxman, A.D. (2006). 'Audit and feedback: Effects on professional practice and healthcare outcomes'. *Cochrane Database of Systematic Reviews,* Issue 2. Art. No.: CD000259. DOI: 10.1002/14651858.CD000259.pub2.

Jorm, A.F., Morgan, A.J. and Hetrick, S.E. (2008). 'Relaxation for depression'.

Cochrane Database of Systematic Reviews. Issue 4. Art. No.: CD007142. DOI: 10.1002/14651858.CD007142.pub2.

Kilo, C.M. (1998). 'A framework for collaborative improvement: Lessons from the Institute for Healthcare Improvement's Breakthrough Series'. *Quality Management in Healthcare*, 6(4), 1–13.

Koenig, H.G. (2008). 'Concerns about measuring "spirituality" in research'. *Journal of Nervous and Mental Disorders*, 196, 349–55.

Koenig, H.G., McCullough, M.E. and Larson, D.B. (2001). *Handbook of Religion and Health*. Oxford: Oxford University Press.

Marie Curie Palliative Care Institute Liverpool (2009). *National Care of the Dying Audit Hospitals Generic Report, 2008/09*. Liverpool: Marie Curie Palliative Care Institute.

Moullin, M. (2002). *Delivering Excellence in Health and Social Care*. Buckingham: Open University Press.

National Institute for Health and Clinical Excellence (2002). *Principles for Best Practice in Clinical Audit*. Oxford: Radcliffe Publishing.

National Institute for Health and Clinical Excellence (2004). *Guidance on Cancer Services: Improving Supportive and Palliative Care for Adults with Cancer*. London: NICE.

National Institute for Health and Clinical Excellence (2007). *Dementia : A NICE–SCIE Guideline on Supporting People with Dementia and their Carers in Health and Social Care*. Leicester: The British Psychological Society.

NHS (2004). *The NHS Knowledge and Skills Framework (NHS, KSF) and the Development Review Process*. London: Department of Health.

NHS Scotland (2008a). *Spiritual Care and Chaplaincy in NHS Scotland, 2008: Revised Guidance, Report and Recommendations*. Glasgow: NHS Educations for Scotland. Available at: http://www.nes.scot.nhs.uk/spiritualcare/ (last accessed April 2010).

NHS Scotland (2008b). *Spiritual and Religious Care Capabilities and Competences for Healthcare Chaplains*. Glasgow: NHS Educations for Scotland. Available at: http://www.nes.scot.nhs.uk/spiritualcare/ (last accessed April 2010).

Øvretveit, J. (2003). *What are the Best Strategies for Ensuring Quality in Hospitals?* Denmark: WHO Regional Office for Europe.

Peterman, A.H., Fitchett, G., Brady, M.J., Hernandez, L. and Cella, D. (2002). Measuring spiritual well-being in people with cancer. *Annals of Behavioural Medicine* 24(1), 49–58.

Royal College of Nursing (2008). *Advanced Nurse Practitioners: An RCN Guide*. London: The Royal College of Nursing.

Scott, T., Mannion, R., Davies, H.T.O. and Marshall, M.N. (2003). 'Implementing culture change in healthcare: Theory and practice'. *International Journal of Quality in Healthcare*, 15(2). 111–18.

Scottish Government (2008). *Living and Dying Well: A National Action Plan for Palliative and End of Life Care in Scotland*. Edinburgh: The Scottish Government.

World Health Organization (2006). *Quality of Care: A Process for Making Strategic Choices in Health Systems*. Geneva: World Health Organization.

Chapter 8
Dilemmas of spiritual assessment

Chris Johnson

Introduction

Apparently John Morton, Lord Chancellor to Henry VII, was a brilliant extractor of forced loans or benevolences, as they were euphemistically called, through what is known as Morton's Fork. His tactic was to go to prominent people and ask them for money. If they were big spenders, then he concluded they must be rich and as such could afford to give money to the King. If on the other hand they spent little, then they must have lots of money hidden away and so could afford to give some to the King. Either way, they were caught on the horns (or the fork!) of a dilemma. Either way, they were the losers.

Dilemmas in the study of spirituality in healthcare abound. This is well illustrated by Mowat (2008, p. 32) who, in her scoping of the literature, lists no less than eighteen themes. Here, I quote just four:

- Nurses should concern themselves with spirituality.
- Nurses should not concern themselves with spirituality.
- There is no need for a definition of spirituality.
- Spirituality can be defined through use of assessment tools.

Leaving aside for a moment 'spiritual assessment', it is not always clear what is meant by assessment in healthcare. What is it that healthcare professionals are assessing?

Assessments in healthcare

Assessments

Health assessments are an essential part of nursing practice. Some nursing historian writers trace the origins back to Florence Nightingale who 'considered assessment as essential nursing function' (Fuller and Schaller-Ayers, 2000, p. 26). She is also reported to have stressed the importance of nursing observation and reporting and the need for nurses to develop technical data-collection skills. Nightingale reputedly emphasised the importance of interviewing patients to gather information about health and illness.

In recent times there has been general agreement about the meaning of nursing assessment. Fuller and Schaller-Ayers (2000, p. 4) define assessment as 'a process of systematically collecting and analyzing data to make judgment about health and life processes of individuals, families and communities'. While emphasising its continuum, Roper *et al.* (1998) view the assessment as the first phase of the process of nursing. Although they recognise some disagreement as to what assessment includes, the following are generally accepted as part of the assessment process:

- collecting information from/about the person
- reviewing the collected information
- identifying the person's problems
- identifying priorities among problems.

The assessment is then followed by three more phases (Roper *et al.*, 1998):

- planning
- implementing, and
- evaluating.

Finally, Fuller and Schaller-Ayer (2000, p.5) warn that it is insufficient for nurse writers to identify areas of nursing care (including spiritual needs) unless assessment areas are described. Citing Black (1967, p.1) they note 'merely saying that the patients had physical, psychological, social and spiritual needs …"fails to point to particulars that are specific enough to guide us in a detailed assessment of needs"'.

Human Needs Model of Nursing

Human Needs Model

Even writers who do not accept Roper *et al.*'s 1998 model of nursing care state 'assessment is the foundation of the nursing process and unless the individual's needs for nursing are deliberately sought, care can never be fully effective' (Minshull *et al.*,

1986, p. 648). Entitling their vision of nursing as the Human Needs Model of Nursing, Minshull *et al.* (1986) base their approach on Maslow's 1954 theory of human needs, arguing that 25 per cent of the nurse's consideration should be given to the physical aspects of care, with equal distribution of emphasis on other categories: safety and security, affiliation needs, dignity and self-esteem and self-actualisation. It is here that perhaps we get close to nursing assessment of spiritual needs.

Thus, although nursing processes may share a common need for patient assessments, the theories may not accommodate the patient's spiritual needs, hence Govier's conclusion (Govier, 2000, p. 34) that 'only a small number of major theorists (Neuman, 1995; Newman, 1989; Parse, 1992: Watson, 1985) identify the spiritual domain in an explicit manner'. Oldnall's opinion (Oldnall, 1995), however, is that 'none actually provides guidelines to help direct the nurse in the process of spiritual assessment' (p. 417).

It is here that the dilemma is realised because it is increasingly assumed (Cobb, 1998; Johnson, 2001) that assessments in spiritual healthcare will take place. But what is meant by 'spiritual care'?

Definition of spiritual care

Definition of spiritual care

The dilemma surrounding a definition of spiritual care that is satisfactory arises from an assumption that both the practitioner and the patient share the same understanding (McSherry, 2004). Clearly this is not so. Writers like Narayanasamy (2002) and Miner-Williams (2006) demonstrate an obvious diversity of definition. It could almost be argued that spirituality is a 'bendy' word; you can make it mean whatever you want depending on the context of usage. Paley (2007, p. 179) describes it as a 'conceptual elastic-band' kind of word. At one extreme writers insist that it can't be used outside a belief in God, while at the other end of the scale it can include 'a concern with fitted kitchens and grouting' (Paley, 2007, p. 179). There are even debates over the most popular of definitions devised by Murray and Zentner (1989; cited in Swinton, 2006) which describes it as 'a quality that goes beyond religious affiliation, that strives for inspiration, reverence, meaning and purpose, even in those who do not believe in any good'. Did their original manuscript say god or good? The literature quotes both, leading to the accusation that if these writers meant good then this suggests there is no necessary ethical content to spirituality, which is unacceptable to many people. For examples, see McSherry and Cash (2003) and Swinton (2006). Swinton (2006, p. 922) rightly ponders other questions such as:

- How did the authors come to this definition?
- What do the components of this definition actually mean?

Various definitions of spiritual care

In my teaching with pre-registration nurses I use various definitions to demonstrate that there is no one way of looking at spirituality in healthcare. I quote the following examples to illustrate my point.

Example 1

The spiritual aspects of patient care are those aspects of human life relating to experiences that transcend sensory phenomena. They are not the same as religious experiences, though for many people religion is an expression of their spirituality. The spiritual dimension of human life may be seen to be holding the physical, psychological and social components. It is often understood as being concerned with meaning and purpose, and for those nearing the end of life it is commonly associated with the need for forgiveness and affirmation of worth.

World Health Organization, 1990, p. 2

Here students sometimes get lost in the words! They ask 'What does transcend sensory phenomena mean?' And 'Why does it just focus on end of life?'

Example 2

It holds together the emotions, convictions and attitudes that charac-terise an individual's life history ... it is the experiential side of religion ... or for those who are not religious, it is an experience of life, that can transport them beyond the mundane ... it is the acknowledgement of a personal significance in the world or sense of uniqueness, of being an individual.

Hammond and Moffitt, 2000, p.2

This extract is long and – just like the WHO – the writers seem to need more words to make their point. Students usually conclude at this point that it is getting so complicated that neither they nor their patients have a chance! No wonder nobody wants to be bothered with spirituality in healthcare!

Example 3

It can refer to the essence of human beings as unique individuals 'what makes me me and you you', so it is the power, energy and hopefulness in a person. It is life at its best, growth and creativity, freedom and love. It is what is deepest in us, what gives us direction, motivation. It is what enables a person to survive bad times ... to overcome difficulties ... to become themselves...

Bradford Social Services, 1999, p. 1

Many students resonate with this definition because (they say) compared to the others it is clear and precise. And that's the dilemma; before patient assessments can be done healthcare professionals have to understand spirituality and what it is they are assessing. One of the problems with this third definition is that it is very individualistic, suggesting spirituality to be something that is 'my affair' so it is impossible to describe and measure. If there are no common threads then how can spirituality be included as part of a nurse's care for the patient?

Reservations about spirituality

Reservations about spirituality

Those who critique the literature on spirituality in healthcare express reservations about spirituality as a concept. In the UK (as distinct from the USA) it is not a word that many find useful. Indeed, many of the students I work with see it as unhelpful. I find myself in agreement with Gilliat-Ray (2003) who finds little evidence of variations of spiritual care appropriate for men, women and children. I would go further and suggest that perhaps there are different spiritualities at different stages of life.

Gilliat-Ray (2003) and Walter (1997; 2002) also state that much of what is defined as spirituality is nothing more than 'psychosocial states of well-being'. Sometimes I have described spirituality as being like an umbrella word for things in life that provide hope, purpose and meaning, such as religious faith, work, pets, family and friends and so on. However, I am inclined to agree with Gilliat-Ray (2003) when she maintains that 'these states of being need to be seen as important in their own right and not part of spirituality' (p. 338). So can we come up with a better word to assist with healthcare assessments? The jury is still out.

Working with those outside healthcare

Working with others

It is my conviction that we are not going to advance the debate around spirituality and assessments until we work with others outside healthcare. Here are two contributions from the sphere of education.

First, citing the Education Act 1988, a paper by NCC Education entitled Spiritual and Moral Development (reprinted by the Schools' Curriculum and Assessment Authority (SCAA), 1995) refers to a dimension of human existence termed the 'spiritual' which applies to all pupils, and also states that 'the potential for spiritual development is open to anyone' (SCAA, 1995, p. 3). The paper discusses many aspects of spiritual development: beliefs, a sense of awe, experience of transcendence, search for meaning and purpose, self-knowledge, relationships, creativity, feelings and emotions. It is interesting to note that the authors are careful not to advocate a linear progression; however they do recognise a development trajectory.

Second, a document produced by the Standing Advisory Committee on Religious Education (SACRE, 1999, p. 4) for North Yorkshire County Council gives guidance for schools on spiritual development and provides the following definition: 'Spiritual is what makes and keeps humans distinctively human'. This is useful in the context of illness and adds a broad dimension for use with all patients. This document further states that characteristically human beings:

- reflect on their own and other's experience, integrating these to make sense of life and their environment; and

- express their sense of meaning and purpose (or lack of it) through spoken and non-spoken forms of communication and the use of symbolism.

These examples provide us with the possibility that if children travel through the education system with a basic understanding of spirituality then perhaps when they reach hospital the confusion over definitions will be considerably less. If on the other hand we have to abandon the use of the word spirituality, as might be necessary, then maybe we will have to substitute spirituality 'sub-words' like hope, meaning and purpose.

Are spiritual assessments possible?

Are spiritual assessments possible?

In the small amount of research done in this area, various systems of spiritual care assessment have been postulated, but it is recognised that these approaches are still in their infancy (Caterall *et al.*, 1988; Cobb, 2001; Labun, 1988; Ross, 1997). However, there are risks attached to 'routinisation of spiritual care'. Walter (2002, p. 137) warns of 'spiritual care' being taken over by the 'flowchart language of the nursing process' and just another patient care compartment, dehumanising the whole process. Likewise McSherry (2001, p. 111) advises caution, saying: 'A danger in constructing and using such tools is that they will reduce assessment of spirituality to a mechanistic or tick-box exercise'.

Similarly, Oldnall argues 'the question must be asked whether or not nurses have the time or education to include spirituality as the fourth domain for the assessment, planning, implementation and evaluation of individualized holistic care' (Oldnall, 1996, p. 417).

Other writers, for example McSherry and Ross (2002, p. 486), maintain that 'it seems there is a need for a systematic review of the available evidence within the area of spiritual assessment' although one of the same researchers elsewhere expresses serious reservations as to whether or not spiritual assessments will ever be possible, because understandings of spirituality are not homogeneous.

Much needs to be done to demonstrate effectiveness of spiritual assessment

Effectiveness of spiritual assessment

We can say therefore that although some work has been done on the effectiveness of spiritual assessment there is much more that needs to be done to *demonstrate* its effectiveness. This uncertainty is possibly because there has been very little research in this area. As Swinton and Narayanasamy (2002) maintain, spirituality is part of what it is to be human and the issue around assessment is due to the lack of confidence and education amongst nurses. Oldnall (1995) and Nolan and Crawford (1997) conclude that nurse education does not prepare nurses adequately to provide spiritual care, and that until the implications of incorporating the language of spirituality into nursing discourse are thoroughly explored, we cannot be certain whether patients are missing out on something that is vital to the integrity of nursing.

Not all patients will have spiritual needs requiring interventions, but it is important for nurses to be aware and sensitive to those needs should they arise (Ross, 1997). Appropriate assessment tools – if they can be found – as part of a care plan, will assist with this process.

Spiritual aspects of healthcare

Spiritual aspects of healthcare

A study of the literature demonstrates a noticeable drive both professionally and politically to establish spirituality as an important and integral part of healthcare provision in the NHS. Reference to spirituality can be found in the following:

- Association of Hospice and Palliative Care Chaplains (2006).
- *Code of Ethics for Nurses* – International Council of Nurses (2000).
- Marie Curie Cancer Care – *Spiritual and Religious Care Competencies for Specialist Palliative Care* (2003).
- Department of Health – *Meeting the Spiritual Needs of Patients and Staff* (1992).
- Department of Health NHS Chaplaincy – *Meeting the Religious and Spiritual Needs of Patients and Staff* (2003).
- *Healthcare Commission Standards* C13a/D2b (Department of Health 2006)
- National Institute for Health and Clinical Excellence (NICE) – *Cancer Care Guidelines (Revised)* (2009).
- Nursing and Midwifery Council – *NMC Code of Professional Conduct* (2004).
- Department of Health – *Patient's Charter* (1991).
- World Health Organization – *Definition of Palliative Care* (2003).
- Department of Health – *Your Guide to the NHS* (2001).

These documents suggest there is a place for spirituality within the context of healthcare; however initiatives such as these have possibly led to false expectations and untested understandings for healthcare workers in the NHS (Orchard, 2001). The implications for staff and the outcomes for patients do not seem to have been seriously considered. Consultation with key stake holders and NHS staff does not appear to have taken place in development of these recommendations. In response, the Department of Health published in 1996 their document *Spiritual Care in the NHS: A Guide for Purchasers and Providers*, in which the authors implied that patients and NHS staff have a clear, shared understanding of what is meant by spiritual care and how it should be delivered to patients.

Two assumptions appear to underline this and other documents (McSherry and Cash, 2003):

● Patients and nurses are aware of their own spiritual needs and comprehend spirituality as presented in healthcare.

● All users of healthcare in the NHS can expect to have their spiritual needs addressed.

More recently the Developmental Standard (D2) of the Healthcare Commission (2007) indicates that 'patients should receive effective treatment and care that takes into account their individual requirements and meets their physical, cultural, spiritual (my italics) and psychological needs and preferences'. Although being a developmental standard it nonetheless is an indicator that for the Department of Health 'spiritual' is understood as an important aspect of healthcare. What then is the purpose of doing spiritual assessments?

Purpose of spiritual assessments

Purpose of spiritual assessments

The National Institute for Health and Clinical Excellence (2004) cancer care guidelines specify 'spiritual care enables individuals and groups to respond to spiritual, emotional and psychological need and to the experience of life, illness and injury, in the context of a personal belief system. Beliefs can be philosophical, religious and/or broadly spiritual in nature' and the Scottish Executive's Spiritual Care in NHS Scotland (Scottish NHS Executive, 2002) states that 'staff should ... be aware of their responsibility for identifying any unmet need and for ensuring that action is taken to address it' (p. 16). Spiritual assessments should therefore be done for the following reasons:

● Because 'person-centred care' is important. In 2005 a joint poster campaign by the NHS, Royal College of Nursing and Help the Aged entitled *See the Person* was designed to remind healthcare staff to see patients 'as people'.

- Because recent models of healthcare have tended to neglect (or misunderstand) spiritual (or religious) needs.

- Because unless these needs are understood and systematically documented then healthcare systems are not treating the 'whole person'.

- Because increasingly patients have high expectations of what the NHS can deliver.

Spiritual assessment is the focus of a discussion by Larry Van de Creek from the USA (2005). He asks many questions including 'Can assessment be insulting to spirituality?' and 'What is a spiritual assessment?'. It must be noted that Van de Creek's understanding of spirituality (he doesn't provide us with a definition) is different to many found in the UK. Essentially spirituality pertains to the patient's relationship to God (or the Sacred) and appears to leave no room for other non-religious approaches to spirituality. Thus he forms a negative question 'Is the relationship to the Sacred something to be used by the person and assessed for its healthcare benefits?'. Clearly the answer is 'No'.

He makes the point that many formats simply screen for spiritual needs; they do not ascertain how spirituality functions in the patient's life. He continues that spiritual screening only identifies *needs*, it does not examine spiritual *function*. Consequently chaplains and other healthcare professionals generally screen for spiritual *needs*, although the process is thought of and described as assessment.

Van de Creek (2005, p. 12) further observes that spiritual screening tools neglect to point out that assessment involves comparing results with an accepted standard. A standard represents the 'normal' or 'healthful'. He draws from medical and nursing assessments and concludes 'whether it is blood pressure or the results of a CT scan, practitioners compare … results to established standards and make diagnostic decisions'.

Van de Creek is right when he maintains there is no spiritual healthcare standard whereby an assessment can be measured. It does not seem to occur to healthcare writers (is there a preoccupation with disease in healthcare?) that it might be good to understand what a spiritually 'well person' looks like. Conversely there is no debate about 'spiritual good health and spiritual bad health'. So maybe there should be a 'gold standard' giving us an idea of what we should all look like! It is left therefore to education to provide us with a starting point. Mackley's (1996) description of what characteristics a spiritually developed person may demonstrate is summarised in Figure 8.1.

Figure 8.1

What a spiritually developed person may be like
(Mackley, 1996).

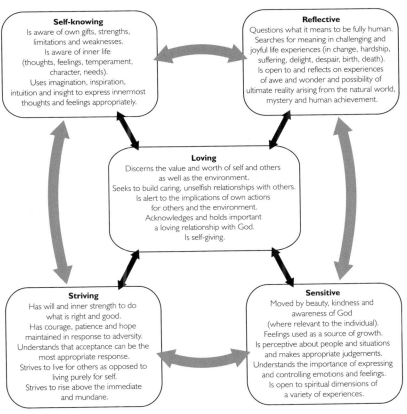

Self-knowing
Is aware of own gifts, strengths, limitations and weaknesses.
Is aware of inner life (thoughts, feelings, temperament, character, needs).
Uses imagination, inspiration, intuition and insight to express innermost thoughts and feelings appropriately.

Reflective
Questions what it means to be fully human.
Searches for meaning in challenging and joyful life experiences (in change, hardship, suffering, delight, despair, birth, death).
Is open to and reflects on experiences of awe and wonder and possibility of ultimate reality arising from the natural world, mystery and human achievement.

Loving
Discerns the value and worth of self and others as well as the environment.
Seeks to build caring, unselfish relationships with others.
Is alert to the implications of own actions for others and the environment.
Acknowledges and holds important a loving relationship with God.
Is self-giving.

Striving
Has will and inner strength to do what is right and good.
Has courage, patience and hope maintained in response to adversity.
Understands that acceptance can be the most appropriate response.
Strives to live for others as opposed to living purely for self.
Strives to rise above the immediate and mundane.

Sensitive
Moved by beauty, kindness and awareness of God (where relevant to the individual).
Feelings used as a source of growth.
Is perceptive about people and situations and makes appropriate judgements.
Understands the importance of expressing and controlling emotions and feelings.
Is open to spiritual dimensions of a variety of experiences.

Spiritual assessment tools

Spiritual assessment tools

There appear to be very few spirituality assessment tools in healthcare in the UK; most are North American and of a religious nature. The context in the US literature mostly relates to cancer care, social work and Chaplaincy. Again dilemmas emerge regarding the difficulties in coming to firm conclusions about the appropriate types of assessment tools.

There are potentially four categories of assessment tools identified through on-line literature searches.

First are patient questionnaires carried out *by nurses* with the patient. These recommend formal assessment for all patients on admission and are used to explore specific patient concerns (Johnson, 2001). However, some patients might consider such in-depth and personal questions offensive and intrusive, especially if they are addressed on admission. These lengthy questionnaires would be almost impossible to use in a hospital acute setting – they are time-consuming and unrealistic. Jones (2004) reminds us that ticks in boxes barely scratch the surface of what is going on in a person's life.

Second are questionnaires completed *by the patients themselves* (self-assessment). They are asked to prioritise their views on meaning, purpose or religion or to score their emotions. Some are based on Likert scales which ask patients how strongly they agree or disagree with various statements. Others are presented as visual analogue scales whereby patients place a cross on a line to indicate their degree of inner conflict. Further models, in contrast to 'problem solving' categories, are designed to support patients in their existing spiritualities and avoid offering inappropriate interventions. However, patients may misunderstand the purpose of these questionnaires, thus leading to confusion between spiritual, religious and psychosocial needs, and resulting in faulty interventions. Although these question-naires can be carried out quickly, they distance the nurse from the patient and can be mechanistic and lack individuality. Also most examples are derived from a Judeo–Christian background (McSherry and Ross, 2002) and as such are inappropriate for patients who do not share these belief systems.

Third are those that relate to the *experiences and instincts* of healthcare professionals. They may use their own experiences, instincts and observations as 'clues' or as a means of identifying patients' spiritual needs. Sometimes they are called indicator-based tools. Also (as indicated in Chapter 4) some healthcare professionals use acronym-based models as aides-memoire to establish during an assessment whether spirituality is a concern to the individual patient.

Fourth are *narrative-based* ones, whereby the patient describes his or her own story. Here, during routine care, the healthcare professional listens as the patient's story unfolds and then identifies any spiritual need or trauma based on his or her 'nursing experiences'. This 'story' is possibly recorded in the patient's documentation to assist with ongoing assessments.

It is noted therefore that three of these (the first, third and fourth) rely on the empathy skills of the healthcare provider, while one (the second) relies on the patient's understanding of spiritual care and knowing their own spiritual needs as they relate to the questionnaire (and may be done with the support and guidance of nurses). As a consequence, Gordon and Mitchell (2004) and the NICE Guidelines (National Institute for Health and Clinical Excellence, 2004) developed competency based skills/levels for staff designed for a palliative care setting. Each of these approaches to assessment has its own capacities but, significantly, Power (2006) observes that 'no one tool has gained widespread acceptance'.

The place of spirituality in healthcare

Spirituality in healthcare

If spiritual healthcare has got a place in modern acute healthcare then it has to substantiate its validity for both patients and staff. In the arena of evidence-based practice, quality healthcare, diagnostic procedures, standardised routines and clinical audit, spirituality is in grave danger of losing its credibility. Cobb (1998) comments that if the spiritual dimension is significant to health and is to be included on the NHS agenda, it will have to demonstrate that it conforms to a health service that is focused on efficiency and effectiveness.

Observing the literature we can conclude that some health professionals (e.g. nurse tutors and chaplains) consider patient spirituality important, while most consider it is not significant enough to be included in 'normal' routine care. Where spiritual assessments are carried out by healthcare staff there are wide discrepancies (for example, nurses' understanding of what is meant by 'spiritual healthcare' and how spiritual care is carried out in practice). My own experience has shown that some staff care spiritually in informal ways, very few are able to articulate the concept, and fewer are competent to document their 'spiritual interventions'. For other staff, 'spiritual' means nothing more than a patient wanting a visit from the hospital imam or going to a Christian chapel service on a Sunday morning. I have spent considerable time looking at patient documentation and observe that occasionally designated space does exist for 'spiritual assessment' (e.g. 'Spiritual, Religious and Psychosocial Assessment') but very rarely is it completed. Staff usually give the following reasons why:

● No time. I'm too busy.

● I don't know what to write.

● I'm not religious.

● Most patients aren't religious.

● Nobody would take any notice of it, even if we did fill it in.

● It should be removed from patient notes.

● It's not the role of nurses – they have too many other things to do.

These comments display a lack of personal confidence and a misunderstanding of the place of spirituality and spiritual needs in healthcare. We must conclude that ways have been tried to raise awareness and assist staff to implement spiritual care, however most have not been very successful in making it a necessary part of patient assessment. True, some have had limited success within small limited specialist areas (like the Liverpool Care Pathway for the Care of the Dying) but no-one has yet devised a generic tool for use across an acute hospital.

Some ethical considerations

Ethical considerations

Patient documentation is an important aspect of the nursing process and a few include sections which cover 'Spiritual needs'. However, some staff have informed me that they do not understand why it is included because a patient's religion is already recorded elsewhere! If it can be argued that documenting spiritual needs is important, then there must be an ethical issue about the content and what (and when) it is recorded (Farvis, 2005). Should there be guidelines for professionals? Is the patient's consent *assumed* as it is with other aspects of nurses' care? Is it just a 'paper exercise' without any possible intervention? In that case, why gather such data?

If the subject of 'spirituality' is explained to patients they may not immediately not recognise any spiritual needs because 'spiritual' has strong religious connotations (McSherry and Draper, 2002). Is it ethical for healthcare teams to provide spiritual healthcare when many do not understand their own spiritualities or if the spiritual care provided is contrary to the healthcare professionals' own spiritual beliefs? Farvis (2005, p. 189) concludes that 'ethical questions … highlight the importance of incorporating the reflective cycle into clinical practice'.

Can any of this be brought together?

Can this be brought together?

Given these numerous dilemmas, very few writers have attempted to bring together aspects from the definitions and rescue something from the pyre. Miner-Williams is one exception. If her approach finds the basis for an understanding of where spirituality fits in within healthcare, then maybe assessment tools can be developed. Here is her thesis (Miner-Williams, 2006, pp. 813–14):

- A person's spirituality is mediated through their values and beliefs, by relational and/or behavioural means.

- The relational manifestation of spirituality is found in the connectedness of relationship (this framework identifies connectedness with 'self', the 'other' (outside of oneself, namely people, animals and nature) or a 'deity').

- The manifestation of spirituality by behavioural means may take place in interactions with others and/or religious practice (and focuses on values such as love, hope, peacefulness, forgiveness and comfort).

- The 'search' is enfolded in 'integrated energy' and the 'transcendent quest' for meaning, purpose and happiness.

- The end focus is health and the alleviation of suffering (where health is defined as wholeness, a unity and harmony of body, mind and spirit).

Miner-Williams (2006, p. 817) draws her argument together in a diagram (Fig. 8.2) to illustrate her point. But Miner-Williams may have fallen once again into the trap of making spirituality in healthcare complicated. She is the first to admit that the challenge is to integrate spirituality into everyday practice and in the context of assessments she falls back on the healthcare practitioner's own experience and instincts model. However, she must be applauded for attempting to make sense of the confusion that seems to exist in this discussion.

Figure 8.2

Transcendent quest for meaning, purpose and happiness

From Miner-Williams (2006) 'Putting a puzzle together: Making spirituality meaningful for nursing using an evolving theoretical framework'. *Journal of Clinical Nursing*, 15(7), 811–21 with kind permission of Wiley-Blackwell Publishing.

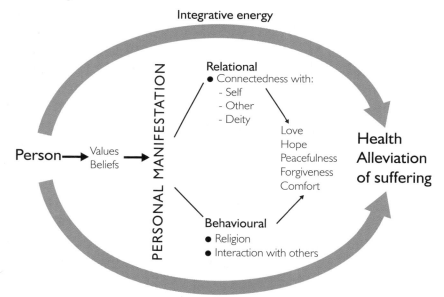

Who should conduct spiritual assessments?

Who should conduct the assessments?

A further question in this debate around spiritual assessments concerns 'Who should conduct them?'. Many nurse theorists, educationalists and practitioners suggest a multidisciplinary approach, with the balance coming down in favour of nurses because 'it is part of nursing practice'. Milligan (2004) maintains that nurses have the edge, but the group least well equipped are medical staff! Nurses are closely followed by chaplains. We note that Van de Creek says that numerous individuals claim spiritual screening and assessment as their professional prerogative, but he argues that they must always be skilled.

Nurses as key players

Nurses are understood therefore as the key players in spiritual care assessment and provision. However, Miner-Williams (2006) argues that they must be at ease with spirituality, of others and of themselves. And she continues that spirituality is about caring for a patient's physical needs as well as the person within. Assessment, therefore, becomes an awareness activity. Caring for your patient means that you get to know them well and are therefore able to pick up the 'cues' about what gives them meaning and happiness, or how they make sense of the illness in their lives.

Similarly Stern and James (2006) develop nurse practice by arguing that nurses must engage with philosophical and religious traditions. In their view education is key to preparing them to give appropriate responses to patients struggling with meaning and meaninglessness.

Walter (2002), Gilliat-Ray (2003) and others are critical of the assumption that all nurses should undertake spiritual care assessment and delivery. Nurses clearly are busy people and perhaps in the current climate too much is expected from them. It is recognised as well (e.g. by Ross, 1994) that many nurses do not feel suitably equipped for the task, even though they may recognise spiritual needs in patients. On the other hand, in an interesting 'interpretive research' article in the *Nursing Standard*, Perry asks 'What contributes to professional fulfilment in nurses?' (Perry, 2005, p. 41). Her work concludes four areas matter to nurses and bring complete satisfaction to their career choice:

- affirming the value of the person
- defending dignity
- enabling hope
- helping patients find meaning.

Even though spirituality is never mentioned, we could legitimately conclude these are all spiritual *values* so perhaps spiritual care is something qualified nurses will continue to do because it is a natural part of caring? Yet it is my experience that in a busy acute hospital healthcare *assistants* may be best placed to spend time with patients and discern their spiritual needs.

Chaplains as part of the assessment process

Considerable progress has been made by the College of Healthcare Chaplains recently, but the dilemma remains for chaplains; they are not healthcare professionals nor are they allied healthcare professionals. This places them in an odd position of having access to patients (with their consent) but being unable professionally to have a significant say in the care of those patients. True, chaplains do make comment, but only when they are invited to do so by healthcare professionals. For most chaplains, unless wards specifically involve them in patient care (e.g. as part of a multidisciplinary team), then it is not possible for assessments to be part of their brief. Chaplains visit patients quite widely and may receive referrals from the patients themselves, from family and friends, from chaplaincy visitors and from healthcare professionals. In a minority of cases a nursing referral may be part of a spiritual assessment, but the majority occur because the patient is religious and a ward 'doesn't know where else to turn'. If, on the other hand, chaplains saw all inpatients then they would be in the ideal position to do assessments, but this would be impractical and unrealistic.

Who should deliver spiritual care?

Who should deliver spiritual care?

One final question remains: If we assume spiritual assessments should be carried out and the findings recorded in care plans, who is the right person to deliver spiritual care? Some consider a variety of people can provide spiritual care, among them are volunteers, family members, social care staff and faith groups (NICE, 2004). However, according to Gilliat-Ray (2003) 'there is a fine line between diagnosis of spiritual need ... and the actual engagement in the delivery of spiritual care'. So are we to conclude that nurses are the only people who can deliver spiritual care? Then if a patient with spiritual distress needs to be 'referred on', who is the appropriate person to refer him or her to? Can we include counsellors, psychologists, or trained volunteers?

Conclusion

In conclusion, the NICE publication *Improving Supportive and Palliative Care for Adults with Cancer* (NICE, 2004, pp. 100–101) concludes that a broad range of professionals may be able to assist individuals with their spiritual needs, if they have the necessary skills and support. Therefore, arguably anyone who can deliver 'skilled, sensitive and appropriate' spiritual care should be encouraged to undertake this. However, NICE (2004) suggest there are four levels of competency, but it is only those achieving Level 3, who are considered capable of *assessing* a patient's spiritual needs by 'developing a plan of care and recognising complex spiritual, religious and ethical needs'. The healthcare professionals at Level 4 are those 'whose primary responsibility is for the spiritual and religious care of patients'. It is interesting to note these recommendations, yet it is still unclear to what extent these competencies and levels are being used in practice.

I remember once discussing these issues with an oncologist. He concluded that if these issues were ever going to be addressed appropriately then each NHS Trust would have to form a 'spiritual care department' (as distinct from a chaplaincy department) that is staffed by professionals drawn from various backgrounds. However, unless there is general agreement on all of these issues then we are a long way off achieving this goal. Some might conclude it will never happen!

References

Association of Hospice and Palliative Care Chaplains (2006). *Standards for Hospice and Palliative Care Chaplaincy*. Glasgow: Help the Hospices.

Black, A. (1967). Cited in J. Fuller and J. Schaller-Ayers (2000). *Health Assessment – A Nursing Approach*. Philadelphia: Lippincott.

Bradford Social Services (1999). *Spiritual Well Being – Policy and Practice. A Working Definition of 'Spiritual'*. Bradford: Bradford Interfaith Education Centre.

Caterall, R., Cox, M., Greet, B., Sankey, J. and Griffiths, G. (1998). 'The assessment and audit of spiritual care'. *International Journal of Palliative Care Nursing*, 4, 162–68.

Cobb, M. (1998). 'Assessing spiritual needs: An examination of practice'. In: M. Cobb and V. Robshaw (eds) *The Spiritual Challenge of Healthcare*. Edinburgh: Churchill Livingstone.

Cobb, M. (2001). *The Dying Soul – Spiritual Care and End of Life*. Buckingham: Oxford University Press.

Department of Health (1991). *Patients Charter*. London: Her Majesty's Stationery Office.

Department of Health (1992). HSG (92)2: *Meeting the Spiritual Needs of Patients and Staff*. London: Her Majesty's Stationery Office.

Department of Health (1996). *Spiritual Care in the NHS. A Guide for Purchasers and Providers*. London: Her Majesty's Stationery Office.

Department of Health (2001). *Your Guide to the NHS*. London: Department of Health.

Department of Health (2003). *NHS Chaplaincy: Meeting the Religious and Spiritual Needs of Patients and Staff*. London: Department of Health.

Department of Health (2006). *Standards for Better Health*. London: Department of Health.

Doble, P. (1999). *SACRE Standing Advisory Committee on Religious Education*. Harrogate: North Yorkshire County Council.

Farvis, R. (2005). 'Ethical considerations in spiritual care'. *Journal of Palliative Nursing*, 11(4), 189.

Fuller, J. and Schaller-Ayers, J. (2000). *Health Assessment – A Nursing Approach*. Philadelphia: Lippincott.

Gilliat-Ray, S. (2003). 'Nursing, professionalism and spirituality'. *Journal of Contemporary Religion*, 18(3), 335–48.

Gordon, T. and Mitchell, D. (2004). 'A competency model for the assessment and delivery of spiritual care'. *Palliative Medicine*, 18, 646–51.

Govier, I. (2000). 'Spiritual care in nursing: A systematic approach'. *Nursing Standard*, 14(17), 32–36.

Hammond, G. and Moffitt, L. (2000). *Spiritual Care – Guidelines for Care Plans*. Leeds: Faith in Elderly People.

Healthcare Commission (2007). *Developmental Standard (D2)*. London: Healthcare Commission.

International Council of Nurses (2000). *Code of Ethics for Nurses*. Geneva: ICN.

Johnson, C. (2001). 'Assessment tools: Are they an effective approach to implementing spiritual healthcare within the NHS?' *Accident and Emergency Nursing*, 9, 177–86.

Jones, L. (2004). 'Practicalities of spiritual assessment. *International Journal of Palliative Nursing*, 10(8), 372.

Labun, E. (1988). 'Spiritual care: An element in nursing care planning. *Journal of Advanced Nursing*, 13, 314–20.

Mackley, J. (1996). 'Characteristics of a spiritually developed person'. *RE Today*, 14(1), 13.

Marie Curie Cancer Care (2003). *Spiritual and Religious Care Competencies for Specialist Cancer Care*. London: Marie Curie.

Maslow, A. (1954). *Motivation and Personality*. New York: Harper and Bros.

McSherry, W. (2001). 'Spiritual crisis: Call a nurse. In: H. Orchard (ed.) *Spirituality in Healthcare Contexts*. London: Jessica Kingsley.

McSherry, W. (2004). *The meaning of spirituality and spiritual care: An investigation of healthcare professionals*. PhD thesis. Leeds Metropolitan University.

McSherry, W. and Cash, K. (2003). 'The language of spirituality'. *International Journal of Nursing Studies*, **41**, 151–61.

McSherry, W. and Draper, P. (2002). 'A critical view of spirituality and spiritual assessment'. *Journal of Advanced Nursing*, **39**(1), 1–2.

McSherry, W. and Ross, L. (2002). 'Dilemmas of spiritual assessment: Considerations for nursing practice'. *Journal of Advanced Nursing*, **38**(5), 479–88.

Milligan, S. (2004). 'Perceptions of spiritual care among nurses undertaking post registration education'. *International Journal of Palliative Nursing*, **10**(4), 162–71.

Miner-Williams, D. (2006). 'Putting a puzzle together: Making spirituality meaningful for nursing using an evolving theoretical framework'. *Journal of Clinical Nursing*, **15**(7), 811–21.

Minshull, J., Ross, K. and Turner, J. (1986). 'The Human Needs model of nursing'. *Journal of Advanced Nursing*, **11**, 643–49.

Mowat, H. (2008). *The Potential for Efficacy of Healthcare Chaplaincy and Spiritual Care Provision in the NHS (UK)*. Aberdeen: Mowat Research, NHS Yorkshire and the Humber.

Murray, R. and Zentner, J. (1989). *Nursing Concepts for Health Promotion*. London: Prentice Hall.

Narayanasamy, A. (2002). 'Spiritual coping mechanisms in chronically ill patients'. *British Journal of Nursing*, **11**(22): 1461–70.

National Institute for Health and Clinical Excellence (2003). *Improving Supportive and Palliative Care for Adults with Cancer – Draft for Second Consultation*. London: National Institute for Health and Clinical Excellence.

Neuman, B. (1995). *The Neuman Systems Model*, 3rd edn. Norwalk: Appleton and Lange.

Newman, M. (1989). 'The spirit of nursing'. *Holistic Nursing Practice*, **3**(3), 1–6.

Nolan, P. and Crawford, P. (1997). 'Towards a rhetoric of spirituality in mental healthcare'. *Journal of Advanced Nursing*, **26**, 289–94.

Nursing and Midwifery Council. (2004). *The NMC Code of Professional Conduct: Standards for Conduct, Performance and Ethics*. NMC: London.

Oldnall, A. (1995). 'On the absence of spirituality in nursing theories and models'. *Journal of Advanced Nursing*, **21**, 417–18.

Oldnall, A. (1996). 'A critical analysis of nursing: meeting the spiritual needs of patients'. *Journal of Advanced Nursing*, **23**, 138–44.

Orchard, H. (2001). *Spirituality in Healthcare Contexts*. Gateshead: Jessica Kingsley.

Paley, J. (2007). 'Spirituality and secularization: Nursing and the sociology of religion'. *Journal of Clinical Nursing*, **17**, 175–86.

Parse, R. (1992). 'Human becoming: Parse's theory of nursing'. *Nursing Science Quarterly*, **5**(1), 35–42.

Perry, B. (2005). 'Core nursing values brought to life through stories'. *Nursing Standard*, **20**(7), 41–48.

Power, J. (2006). 'Spiritual assessment: Developing an assessment tool'. *Nursing Older People*, 18(2), 16–19.

Roper, N., Logan, W. and Tierney, A. (1998). *The Elements of Nursing*, 4th edn. London: Churchill Livingstone.

Ross, L. (1994). 'Spiritual care: The nurse's role'. *Nursing Standard*, 8(29): 35–37.

Ross, L. (1997). *Nurses' Perceptions of Spiritual Care*. Aldershot, Avebury.

Schools' Curriculum and Assessment Authority (1995). *Spiritual and Moral Development. Discussion Paper No.3*. London: National Curriculum Council.

Scottish NHS Executive (2002). *Spiritual Care in NHS Scotland*. Edinburgh: Scottish Executive.

Stern, J. and James, S. (2006). 'Every person matters: Enabling spirituality education for nurses'. *Journal of Clinical Nursing*, 15, 897–904.

Swinton, J. (2006). 'Identity and resistance: Why spiritual care needs "enemies"'. *Journal of Clinical Nursing*, 15(7), 918–28.

Swinton, J. and Narayanasamy, A. (2002). 'Response to: "A critical view of spirituality and spiritual assessment" by P. Draper and W. McSherry'. *Journal of Advanced Nursing*, 40(2), 158–60.

Van de Creek, L. (2005). 'Spiritual assessment: Six questions and an annotated bibliography'. *Chaplaincy Today*, 21(1), 11–15.

Walter, T. (1997). 'The ideology and organization of spiritual care'. *Palliative Medicine*, 11, 21–30.

Walter, T. (2002). 'Spirituality in palliative care: Opportunity or burden?' *Palliative Medicine*, 16, 133–39.

Watson, J. (1985). *Nursing: The Philosophy and Science of Caring*. Boulder, CO: Colorado Association University Press.

World Health Organization (1990). *WHO Definition of Spiritual Healthcare*. Geneva: WHO.

World Health Organization (2003). *WHO Definition of Palliative Care*. Geneva: WHO.

Chapter 9
Considerations for the future of spiritual assessment
Linda Ross and Wilfred McSherry

Introduction

This chapter reflects upon the challenges that still surround spiritual assessment and highlights considerations for its future development. The editors and many of the contributors to this book have undertaken a great deal of scholarship and research in the area of spirituality, spanning several decades. Despite all this activity the evidence presented here suggests there has been no significant change in the area. The spiritual dimension is still not formally integrated within the philosophy and culture of healthcare. In some countries, the concept is still very much on the periphery of healthcare practice. However, there are some promising signs, for example a shift from a purely medical reductionist model of healthcare to one that acknowledges the importance of personal beliefs and values for the health and well-being of individuals. Yet, despite decades of activity directed at the spiritual dimension, many healthcare practitioners still feel uncomfortable and ill-prepared to assess and support patients/clients in this fundamental area, and this raises the question why? This chapter, therefore, offers a Model for Actioning Spiritual Care. The model provides a framework that may enable some of the challenges to be overcome so that practitioners are prepared for assessing and providing spiritual care within diverse caring settings.

Spectrum of beliefs

Spectrum of beliefs

As outlined earlier in this text one of the main considerations when designing any form of spiritual assessment is the notion of inclusivity. Inclusivity in this context means that the tools are sensitive to the full spectrum of people's beliefs, i.e. to people who have a spiritual or religious belief and those who do not. Therefore, healthcare must listen to the voice and concerns of all in society. Some small sections of society are very vocal and proactive, but this does not mean that their criticisms and opposition are necessarily in the best interests of all. Their arguments and objections may be based on a distorted and immature insight into some very complex debates. We would recommend that anyone developing spiritual assessment tools ensures that there is broad representation to capture the full spectrum of beliefs and that service users are consulted at every stage of the construction and evaluation. This level of inclusivity and objectivity will ensure tools are fit for purpose and for the healthcare context.

'Silo' working

'Silo' working

When one reviews the development of spiritual assessment across the healthcare professions it is noticeable that (up until recently) there has been a lack of collaboration and cooperative working. By this we mean the sharing of innovative ideas and practices that can be modelled or adopted by others. Each discipline adopts a 'silo' mentality, constructing and discussing the implications of spiritual assessment within the constraints and boundaries of their own professional practice. It could be argued that this is necessary because spiritual assessment tools used in social work or family therapy will incorporate strategies that may not be suitable for nurses admitting patients onto acute hospital wards. Yet despite the different contexts there are many principles relating to design and usage that could be shared. Evidence is emerging to show that different professions are now working with each other in the construction and utilisation of spiritual assessment strategies.

Integrated care

Integrated care

A potential dilemma of focusing specifically upon spiritual assessment is that practitioners may see it as a separate and discrete area of assessment. Spiritual care may then become fragmented, reducing the individual into another category. People may be viewed as 'parts' and spiritual need becomes another box to be ticked or another assessment to be undertaken. This approach to spiritual care is divisive. Rather, spiritual care should be seen as integral to the caring process. Spiritual care is often hidden – it is often the intuitive aspects of care and caring. Therefore, if spiritual assessment is not carefully planned and designed then there is the potential to complicate care. By this we mean that spiritual care is made out to be something complex and difficult, when in reality many healthcare professionals are already providing spiritual care, without actually labelling it as such. Bradshaw's seminal work (Bradshaw, 1994, p. 282) stresses the importance of integration: 'Physical care therefore brings with it spiritual care. And spiritual care is inseparable from physical, social and psychological care because it is indistinguishable from the wholeness of care'.

Spiritual care for all

Spiritual care for all

Before we can action spiritual care there must be some exploration as to whether spiritual care is legitimate for all. Healthcare professionals cannot and should not make assumptions about what patients want and expect in this area. Not all patients entering healthcare will present with a spiritual or religious need. Therefore, is it ethical to routinely enquire and assess all patients for potential spiritual needs? The solution is to always be guided by the patient. If they should express a need in this area then intervention may be necessary. Perhaps one way of approaching this question is to reflect upon the following approaches – practitioner-led or expressed need? Subjecting patients to routine spiritual assessment may be, as one charge nurse implied, over-stepping the mark:

> *We are not here to take over that person, we are not here to encroach on what they think or do. We are here to cut out their in-growing toe nail or whatever sometimes, and that is what people want. We haven't got that right, to worm our way to that patient's thoughts, unless of course they want us to. We have no right to do that. I would object. I sometimes think we are too familiar with people, we shouldn't expect to be.*
>
> McSherry, 2007

Actioning spiritual care

At the end of the day the most important thing is that patients' spiritual needs are recognised and met or supported, hence this is at the heart of our Model for Actioning Spiritual Care using a systematic approach (Fig. 9.1). This model builds upon our previous work in which we suggested the use of the *nursing process* as a systematic method for ensuring that spiritual needs are assessed and care planned, implemented and evaluated in order to ensure that spiritual needs are met and sustained (Ross, 1997b). We used the term *nursing process* at that time. We have simply called it a *systematic approach* here because the same four steps can be applied to any discipline. Many factors related to the healthcare practitioner and the environment will influence how the process works in practice, but it is important that the patient takes the lead, that the process is guided and directed by them as part of person-centred care (lower part of Fig. 9.1).

Figure 9.1   **Model for actioning spiritual care using a systematic approach.**

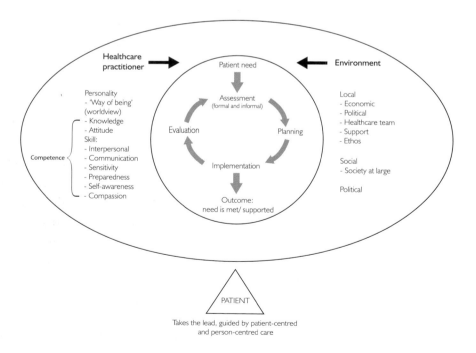

Importance of assessment

Importance of assessment

The first step in the actioning of spiritual care is the assessment (central part of Fig. 9.1). Unless an assessment is undertaken none of the other stages (planning, intervention and evaluation) will happen, and patients' spiritual needs will be ignored. This is why we feel this book is especially important. Many tools and approaches to spiritual assessment and their associated dilemmas have been discussed in Chapters 4, 5 and 7 but it is unlikely that any one will serve as a magic wand to ensure that patients' spiritual needs are recognised and met or supported. Rather it is probably more about increasing healthcare professionals' awareness of and sensitivity to the spiritual dimension, so that they can pick up on the cues that patients display and respond using whichever tools and skills (having a range of options to hand would probably help) are most appropriate at that moment in time (Chapter 3). This process of picking up on cues (assessment) and responding (planning and intervention) will be dynamic and constantly changing (as indicated by the circular movement of the arrows on Fig. 9.1) so it is unlikely that one rigid form of assessment will fit.

How exactly we prepare healthcare professionals for such a role is not yet clear and it remains the subject of debate and enquiry (for example, see Maben and Griffiths, 2008). Clearly a certain degree of knowledge is required (left-hand side of Fig. 9.1). Thus it would be important for nurses to be aware of evidence about the influence of belief and faith on health outcomes (some of the measures and tools used in this research are discussed in Chapter 6), and the evidence within nursing about the practice of spiritual care, as well as the types of assessment tools available, and so on. However, it is not just about the knowledge possessed by the healthcare professional but also about their own skills and attitudes – that is, their competency (left-hand side of Fig. 9.1).

In our research with patients and nurses it is clear that patients very quickly decide which nurse is approachable and which is not; the nurse's 'way of being' or 'personality' and worldview seems to be important (Ross, 1997a, 1997b). For example one patient commented: 'there are always those who are more helpful than others. Some can't do enough. Others screw up their faces when you ask them. They're happy people … there's one in particular. She couldn't have chosen a better occupation for herself if she'd tried'.

And another stated: 'the ones that are helpful … it's their personality and the way they deal with a situation. It's something that's difficult to explain but you know very quickly…' (Ross, 1997a, p. 713).

Quality of carers

The challenge is how we produce healthcare professionals with that 'personality' or perhaps a 'way of being' that patients would seem to value. What skills and attitudes make up that 'way of being'? Our previous research (and that by others since) highlights the importance of interpersonal/communication skills, sensitivity and preparedness/self-awareness (Ross, 1997b). The healthcare professional's own personal spirituality, beliefs and values will also enter the equation, as discussed in Chapter 2. Compassion would also seem to feature highly. One of the essential skills clusters identified by the Nursing and Midwifery Council is for 'care, compassion and communication' whereby 'patients/clients can trust a newly registered nurse to: provide care that is delivered in a warm, sensitive and compassionate way' (Nursing and Midwifery Council, 2007, p. 4). Smiling and being cheerful are characteristics patients use to measure a caring nurse, according to Ford (2009). But how can we foster the acquisition of these skills and attitudes which, when combined with knowledge, produce healthcare professionals who are competent in delivering spiritual care at point of registration (a requirement of the Nursing and Midwifery Council and the Quality Assurance Agency for Higher Education). These are questions that both the NMC and Quality Assurance Agency for Higher Education (QAAHE) are currently investigating through research.

The formal and informal

Having said that the process of assessing and responding to spiritual needs will be dynamic and that no single tool or approach is likely to suffice, the authors of this chapter would however advocate some sort of formal assessment on admission to identify any religious or non-religious practices that may be of particular importance to the patient. We make this suggestion because of our experience in caring for patients and their families in our clinical work. We have both encountered situations in which patients and their families have been exposed to unnecessary distress because essential information about their religious beliefs and practices were not documented on admission (e.g. see Peter's case in McSherry, 2006, pp. 108–09). While our experience has related to religious beliefs and practices it is possible that people with no religious faith may have beliefs and practices that are important to them, so it would be equally important that these are documented on admission. Therefore, spiritual assessment should perhaps include both formal elements (on admission) and informal elements (ongoing after admission).

Having completed the assessment, care can then be planned, implemented and evaluated, again with the patient taking the lead.

Of course factors in the local and wider environment will also impact upon whether spiritual care is given and how it is given (Ross, 1997b) (see right-hand side of Fig. 9.1). Locally, political decisions and the economic climate will influence the type of service that can be offered. The ambience and ethos will also be influential factors, as will the dynamics and level of support within the healthcare team. Some of these factors will in turn be influenced by decisions and policies made at worldwide, European and country-wide levels. Chapters 1 and 8 explore these aspects in some detail. Of course society changes over time too, and policy must respond if it is to continue to meet the true needs of a country's population. For example, the NHS chaplaincy guidance document was altered in 2000 to better serve the needs of an increasingly religiously diverse society (Department of Health, 2003). This document seems to have been superseded by the publication of *Religion and Belief* (Department of Health, 2009). Again this document highlights the importance of personal and religious beliefs, while emphasising the need for sensitivity and self-awareness in the provision of healthcare.

Art and science

Art and science

There would seem to be a need to balance the 'art' (those humanistic qualities of care and caring such as communication) and 'science' (concerns with treatment and technical competence, measurement and outcome) within spiritual care (Fig. 9.2). Both sides of the scale are of equal importance if equilibrium is to be restored and achieved in healthcare practice. The imbalance is evident in this statement made during an interview by one terminally ill patient:

'Wilf, we get treatment in the hospital and care in the hospice'.

This phrase has significance and poignancy within the context of today's healthcare system. The fact that this gentleman was able to make a distinction between 'treatment' and 'care' strikes at the heart of some of the issues that are impacting upon various healthcare sectors. The phrase implies 'treatment' is different to 'care'. It highlights the importance of balance in the delivery of healthcare, and has direct relevance for the area of spiritual assessment. The scale must balance. If it tips too much towards the artistic side then tools may lack rigour. If it tips too much towards the scientific side then tools may fail to engage or capture the humanistic elements of spiritual care. Such tools may not be person-centred and sensitive to the needs of the individual.

Figure 9.2   **The need for balance in spiritual care.**
Re-discovery of a forgotten dimension

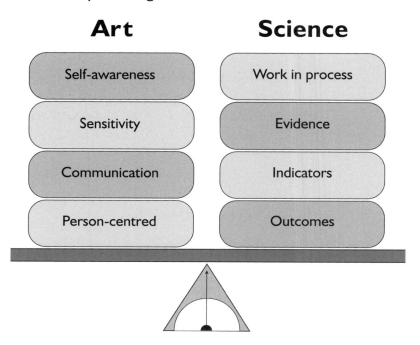

Over the last three decades the concept of spirituality has grown in popularity within both society and healthcare. We would now argue that despite recent criticism it is recognised as a crucial and central dimension of people's lives. Swinton (2001) referred to spirituality as re-discovering a 'forgotten' dimension. Within the UK there have been a growing number of reports about people who are subjected to neglect and abuse within healthcare organisations (Healthcare Commission, 2009; The Patients Association, 2009). What is noticeable and a recurrent theme in these documents is the perceived erosion of care and caring. Patients and families tell of staff who did not treat them with dignity and respect, describing how they were denied the fundamentals of care. They argue that the core values that once underpinned healthcare practice have vanished. Such reports indicate that healthcare practitioners do not have the time to care. There seems to be an over-emphasis on outcome measures, budgets, and financial targets. We would argue that the time is now right to re-discover and re-invest in the spiritual dimension. By re-focusing on the spiritual, many of the problems that have been reported will be rectified because care will once again focus upon the individual.

There are some very positive and encouraging signs with regards to the spiritual dimension of healthcare. For example the National Health Service in Scotland has developed policy and guidance highlighting the importance of spiritual care (NHS Education for Scotland, 2009).

> *The provision of spiritual care by NHS staff is not yet another demand on their hard-pressed time. It is the very essence of their work and it enables and promotes healing in the fullest sense to all parties, both giver and receiver, of such care.*
>
> NHS Education for Scotland, 2009, p. 4

Conclusion

We began this chapter by reflecting on the fact that what we seemed to be writing was reminiscent of our work almost two decades ago and asking ourselves if anything had changed in that time. There is undoubtedly greater recognition of the importance of the spiritual part of life health and well-being today compared with 10 or 20 years ago. This is evidenced by the number of policy and guidance documents that have emerged in recent years. There has also been an increasing evidence base, not only in the health outcomes research which demonstrates a strong link between faith/belief and health/well-being (e.g. Koenig *et al.*, 2001) but also in research into the patients' and healthcare professionals' perceptions and experience of spiritual needs and care (e.g. Ross, 2006). Considerable work has also focused upon the development of spiritual assessment and audit tools.

However, coming back to the person central to our healthcare system – the patient – we have to ask: What has actually changed in practice? Is the patient's experience any different? Is the spiritual part of the patient actually catered for routinely as part of his or her care package? The answers to these questions are by no means clear.

On the one hand, we hear of examples of excellence in holistic care, usually within the palliative care setting as illustrated by the patient's comment above. But there are also concerning reports, as previously mentioned, of instances in which care and compassion have been absent and dignity has not been respected. If all was well and patients were being cared for in a holistic and dignified manner, then why did the Royal College of Nursing feel the need to launch its dignity campaign with the slogan 'Dignity – at the heart of everything we do' (Royal College of Nursing, 2008)?. Sadly there is plenty to indicate that spiritual care may not be happening in practice. To that end we offer a model for actioning spiritual care so that it becomes, in the words of the National Health Service for Scotland, 'the very essence of' our 'work'. We hope that the model is a useful tool in that respect, so that all patients – not just those receiving palliative care – are assisted to achieve an optimum state of physical, mental, social and spiritual well-being.

References

Bradshaw, A. (1994). *Lighting the Lamp. The Spiritual Dimension of Nursing Care.* London: Scutari Press.

Department of Health (2003). *NHS Chaplaincy. Meeting the Religious and Spiritual Needs of Patients and Staff.* London: Department of Health.

Department of Health (2009). *Religion and Belief*. London: Department of Health.

Ford, S. (2009). 'Patients view smiling as best indicator of nurse skill'. Available at: www.nursingtimes.net/whats-new-in-nursing/acute-care/patients-view-smiling-as-best-indicator-of-nurse-skill/5006094.article (last accessed April 2010)

Healthcare Commission (2009). *Investigation into Mid Staffordshire NHS Foundation Trust Commission for Healthcare Audit and Inspection*. London: Healthcare Commission.

Koenig, H.G., Larson, D.B. and McCullough, M.E. (2001). *Handbook of Religion and Health*. New York: Oxford University Press.

Maben, J. and Griffiths, P. (2008). *Nurse in Society: Starting the Debate*. London: Kings College.

McSherry, W. (2006). *Marking Sense of Spirituality in Nursing and Healthcare Practice: An Interactive Approach*, 2nd edn. London: Jessica Kingsley.

McSherry, W. (2007). *The Meaning of Spirituality and Spiritual Care within Nursing and Healthcare Practice*. London: Quay Books.

NHS Education for Scotland (2009). *Spiritual Care Matters. An Introductory Resource for all NHS Scotland Staff*. Edinburgh: NES.

Nursing and Midwifery Council (2007). *Essential Skills Clusters (ESCs) for Pre-Registration Nursing Programmes*. NMC Circular 07/2007. London: NMC.

Ross, L. (1997a). 'Elderly patients' perceptions of their spiritual needs and care: A pilot study'. *Journal of Advanced Nursing*, **26**, 710–15.

Ross, L. (1997b). *Nurses' Perceptions of Spiritual Care*. Aldershot: Avebury.

Ross, L. (2006). 'Spiritual care in nursing: An overview of the research to date'. *Journal of Clinical Nursing*, **15**(7), 852–62.

Royal Collage of Nursing (2008). 'RCN launches major campaign on dignity'. *RCN Bulletin*, **204**, 1.

Swinton, J. (2001). *Spirituality and Mental Healthcare: Re-Discovering a 'Forgotten' Dimension*. London: Jessica Kingsley.

The Patients Association (2009). *Patients Not Numbers . People Not Statistics*. London: The Patients Association.

Useful websites

British Association for the Study of Spirituality (BASS)
http://www.basspirituality.org.uk

George Washington Institute for Spirituality and Health (GWish)
http://www.gwish.org

NHS Core Principles
http://www.nhs.uk/NHSEngland/aboutnhs/Pages/NHSCorePrinciples.aspx

Nursing Times
http://www.nursingtimes.net

Royal College of Psychology
http://www.rcpsych.ac.uk/spirit

Scottish Executive guidelines on chaplaincy and spiritual care
http://www.nes.scot.nhs.uk/spiritualcare

Spirituality in the workplace
http://www.workplacespirituality.org.uk

World Health Organization
http://www.who.int/en

Index